Oxford Case Histories
in Oncology

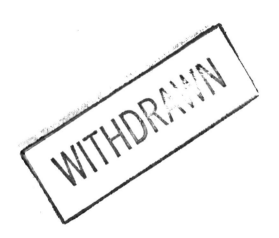

Oxford Case Histories

Series Editors:

Sarah Pendlebury and Peter Rothwell

Published:

Neurological Case Histories (Sarah Pendlebury, Philip Anslow, and Peter Rothwell)

Oxford Case Histories in Cardiology (Rajkumar Rajendram, Javed Ehtisham, and Colin Forfar)

Oxford Case Histories in Gastroenterology and Hepatology (Alissa Walsh, Otto Buchel, Jane Collier, and Simon Travis)

Oxford Case Histories in Respiratory Medicine (John Stradling, Andrew Stanton, Najib Rahman, Annabel Nickol, and Helen Davies)

Oxford Case Histories in Rheumatology (Joel David, Anne Miller, Anushka Soni, and Lyn Williamson)

Oxford Case Histories in TIA and Stroke (Sarah Pendlebury, Ursula Schulz, Aneil Malhotra, and Peter Rothwell)

Oxford Case Histories in Neurosurgery (Harutomo Hasegawa, Matthew Crocker, and Pawan Singh Minhas)

Oxford Case Histories in Oncology (Thankamma Ajithkumar, Adrian Harnett, and Tom Roques)

Oxford Case Histories in Oncology

Edited by

Thankamma Ajithkumar

Adrian Harnett

Tom Roques

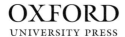

OXFORD
UNIVERSITY PRESS

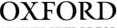

OXFORD
UNIVERSITY PRESS

Great Clarendon Street, Oxford, OX2 6DP,
United Kingdom

Oxford University Press is a department of the University of Oxford.
It furthers the University's objective of excellence in research, scholarship,
and education by publishing worldwide. Oxford is a registered trade mark of
Oxford University Press in the UK and in certain other countries

First Edition published in 2014

Impression: 1

Published in the United States of America by Oxford University Press
198 Madison Avenue, New York, NY 10016, United States of America

British Library Cataloguing in Publication Data

Data available

Library of Congress Control Number: 2013949003

ISBN 978–0–19–966453–5

Printed and bound in Great Britain by
CPI Group (UK) Ltd, Croydon, CR0 4YY

A note from the series editors

Case histories have always had an important role in medical education, but most published material has been directed at undergraduates or residents. The Oxford Case Histories series aims to provide more complex case-based learning for clinicians in specialist training and consultants, with a view to aiding preparation for entry- and exit-level specialty examinations or revalidation.

Each case book follows the same format with approximately 50 cases, each comprising a brief clinical history and investigations, followed by questions on differential diagnosis and management, and detailed answers with discussion.

At the end of each book, cases are listed by mode of presentation, aetiology, and diagnosis. We are grateful to our colleagues in the various medical specialties for their enthusiasm and hard work in making the series possible.

Sarah Pendlebury and Peter Rothwell

From reviews of other books in the series:

Neurological Case Histories
'...contains 51 cases that cover the spectrum of acute neurology and the neurology of general medicine—this breadth makes the volume unique and provides a formidable challenge...it is a heavy-duty diagnostic series of cases, and readers have to work hard, to recognise the diagnosis and answer the questions that are posed for each case...I recommend this excellent volume highly...'

Lancet Neurology

'This short and well-written text is...designed to enhance the reader's diagnostic ability and clinical understanding...A well-documented and practical book.'

European Journal of Neurology

Oxford Case Histories in Gastroenterology and Hepatology
'...a fascinating insight into clinical gastroenterology, an excellent and enjoyable read and an education for all levels of gastroenterologist from ST1 to consultant.'

Gut

Preface

Oncology is one of the most rapidly changing specialties due to the continuing development of new therapies and technologies. The combination of basic principles of clinical practice with these new tools is often challenging for both experienced clinicians and trainees. Textbooks are narratives of facts which are useful for learning the established principles of clinical management, but in the real situation it is a quite different story when the patient is sitting in front of you, a far more interesting but also far more challenging proposition. Case studies make the background knowledge real and applicable. They are thought-provoking and help to improve critical thinking and interpretive skills.

The design of this book is to challenge you to make appropriate evidence-based management decisions in a wide range of real clinical scenarios. The cases in this book cover a wide spectrum of oncology and include both uncommon presentations and clinical problems of common cancers, and various challenges which occur from time to time with uncommon cancers. We hope that these cases will help you to confidently apply the basic principles and latest evidence in clinical decision-making. Each case comprises a short history followed by questions and answers. The answers are based on the latest clinical research, systematic reviews, meta-analyses, and guidelines from national and international associations (including the National Institute of Health and Care Excellence, the Scottish Intercollegiate Guidelines Network, the American Society of Clinical Oncology, and the European Society of Medical Oncology).

We hope this book will be an essential tool for many, including non-specialist readers, clinicians in oncology and palliative care, specialist nurses, radiographers, and other members of the multidisciplinary team. Most of all, and unlike a textbook, we hope that you find this book entertaining and that it stimulates you to move on in the care for your patients in order to give them the very best.

T. Ajithkumar, A. Harnett, T. Roques
2013

Acknowledgements

We are thankful to Professor Ann Barrett for her guidance and editorial comments. We are grateful to Nicola Wilson and Caroline Smith at Oxford University Press for commissioning this book and supporting us throughout its development and production.

Contents

Abbreviations

ABVD	adriamycin, bleomycin, vinblastine, and dacarbazine	**DFS**	disease-free survival
		DRE	digital rectal examination
AED	antiepileptic drug	**DTIC**	dacarbazine
AFP	α-fetoprotein	**EC**	endometrioid carcinoma
AJCC	American Joint Committee on Cancer	**ECF**	epirubicin, cisplatin, and 5-fluorouracil
ALK	anaplastic lymphoma kinase	**ECOG**	Eastern Cooperative Oncology Group
ALT	alanine aminotransferase	**ECX**	epirubicin, cisplatin, and capecitabine
ARMS	alveolar rhabdomyosarcoma	**EGFR**	epidermal growth factor receptor
AST	aspartate aminotransferase		
BCCA	British Columbia Cancer Agency	**EMA**	epithelial membrane antigen
BEP	bleomycin, etoposide, and cisplatin	**ENETS**	European Neuroendocrine Tumor Society
BHD	Birt–Hogg–Dubé [syndrome]	**EOC**	epithelial ovarian cancer
		EQD2	2Gy equivalent doses
BSO	bilateral salpingo-oophorectomy	**ER**	oestrogen
		EUA	evaluation/examination under general anaesthesia
CA	cancer antigen		
cAMPK	cellular-activated mitogen protein kinase	**EUS**	endoscopic ultrasound
		FBC	full blood count
CCC	clear cell carcinoma	**FDA**	(US) Food and Drug Administration
cCR	complete clinical response		
CDX2	caudal type homeobox 2	**¹⁸FDG PET-CT**	fluorine-18 fluorodeoxyglucose positron emission tomography–computed tomography
CEA	carcinoembryonic antigen		
ChRCC	chromophobe renal cell carcinoma		
CK	cytokeratin	**FEC**	5-fluorouracil, epirubicin, and cyclophosphamide
CRM	circumferential resection margin	**FIGO**	International Federation of Gynecology and Obstetrics
CSF	cerebrospinal fluid		
CT	computed tomography		
CTV	clinical target volume	**FISH**	fluorescence *in situ* hybridization
DCIS	ductal carcinoma *in situ*	**5-FU**	5-fluorouracil

GCDFP-15	gross cystic disease fluid protein-15
GI	gastrointestinal
GIST	gastrointestinal stromal tumour
GTV	gross tumour volume
HAART	highly active antiretroviral therapy
β-hCG	beta human chorionic gonadotropin
HGS	high-grade serous
5-HIAA	5-hydroxyindoleacetic acid
HPF	high-power field
HPV	human papillomavirus
HR	hazard ratio
IARC	International Agency for Research on Cancer
ICRU	International Commission on Radiation Units and Measurements
IGBT	image-guided brachytherapy
IGCCCG	International Germ Cell Cancer Collaborative Group
IT	intrathecal
LCNEC	large cell neuroendocrine carcinoma
LDH	lactate dehydrogenase
LGS	low-grade serous (carcinoma)
LHRH	luteinizing hormone releasing hormone
MAP	cisplatin with doxorubicin and high-dose methotrexate
MCC	Merkel cell carcinoma
MDT	multidisciplinary team
MEN	multiple endocrine neoplasia
MRF	mesorectal fascia
MRI	magnetic resonance imaging
MSKCC	Memorial Sloan-Kettering Cancer Center

mTOR	mammalian target of rapamycin complex
NCI	National Cancer Institute
NICE	National Institute for Health and Care Excellence
NIH	National Institutes of Health
NSCLC	non-small cell lung cancer
NSGCT	non-seminomatous germ cell tumour
OAR	organ at risk
ORR	overall response rate
OS	overall survival
PARP	poly-ADP ribose polymerase
PASH	pseudo-angiomatoid stromal hyperplasia
PCI	prophylactic cranial irradiation
PCR	polymerase chain reaction
PET	positron emission tomography
PFS	progression-free survival
PgR	progesterone
PLAP	placenta-like alkaline phosphatase
PSA	prostate-specific antigen
PTV	planning target volume
RCC	renal cell carcinoma
RMI	risk of malignancy index
SCLC	small cell lung cancer
SREs	skeletal-related events
SSIGN score	stage, size, grade, and necrosis score
TAH	total abdominal hysterectomy
TCX	trastuzumab, cisplatin, and capecitabine
TKI	tyrosine kinase inhibitor
TNM	tumour, node, metastasis
TTF-1	thyroid transcription factor 1
U&Es	urea and electrolytes

UISS	UCLA integrated staging system	**VEGF**	vascular endothelial growth factor
UKI NETS	UK and Ireland Neuroendocrine Tumour Society	**WART**	whole abdominal radiotherapy
US	ultrasound	**WHO**	World Health Organization

List of contributors

Thankamma Ajithkumar
Consultant Clinical Oncologist
Norfolk and Norwich University
Hospital
Norwich, UK

Susanna Alexander
Consultant Medical Oncologist
Norfolk and Norwich University
Hospital
Norwich, UK

Oliver Bassett
Research Fellow in Melanoma
Mount Vernon Cancer Centre
Middlesex, UK

Bristi Basu
Cancer Research UK Consultant Medical
Oncologist and Academic Consultant in
Experimental Cancer Therapeutics
Cambridge University Hospitals NHS
Trust
Cambridge, UK

Debashis Biswas
Consultant Clinical Oncologist
Norfolk and Norwich University
Hospital
Norwich, UK

Sara Custodio-Cabello
Clinical Oncology Resident
Hospital General Universitario Gregorio
Marañon,
Madrid, Spain

Spyridon Gennatas
Specialist Registrar in Medical Oncology
Royal Marsden Hospital
London, UK

Michael Gonzalez
Senior Clinical Fellow
The Royal Marsden NHS Foundation
Trust
London, UK

Ioannis Gounaris
Specialist Registrar in Medical Oncology
Cambridge University Hospitals NHS
Trust
Cambridge, UK

Adrian Harnett
Consultant Clinical Oncologist
Norfolk and Norwich University
Hospital
Norwich, UK

Helen Hatcher
Consultant in Medical and TYA
Oncology
Cambridge University Hospitals NHS
Trust
Cambridge, UK

Nicola Holtom
Consultant in Palliative Medicine
Norfolk and Norwich University
Hospital
Norwich, UK

Simon Johnston
Academic Clinical Fellow in Medical
Oncology
Addenbrooke's Hospital, Cambridge, UK

Gaurav Kapur
Consultant Clinical Oncologist
Norfolk and Norwich University
Hospital
Norwich, UK

Khurum Khan
Clinical Research Fellow
The Royal Marsden NHS Foundation
Trust
London, UK

Elizabeth Liniker
Academic Clinical Fellow in Medical
Oncology
Addenbrooke's Hospital, Cambridge, UK

Suat W. Loo
Consultant Clinical Oncologist
Norfolk and Norwich University
Hospital
Norwich, UK

Isabella Maund
Specialist Registrar in Clinical Oncology
Cambridge University Hospitals NHS
Trust

Paul Nathan
Consultant Medical Oncologist
Director, Research and Development
Mount Vernon Cancer Centre
Middlesex, UK

Jenny Nobes
Consultant Clinical Oncologist
Norfolk and Norwich University
Hospital
Norwich, UK

Christine Parkinson
Consultant Medical Oncologist
Cambridge University Hospitals NHS
Trust
Cambridge, UK

Sanjay Popat
Clinical Senior Lecturer, Imperial
College, London and Consultant Medical
Oncologist, Royal Marsden Hospital
London, UK

Federica Recine
Department of Medical Oncology
San Camillo and Forlanini Hospital
Rome, Italy

Tom Roques
Consultant Clinical Oncologist
Norfolk and Norwich University
Hospital
Norwich, UK

Cora Sternberg
Chief
Department of Medical Oncology
San Camillo Forlanini Hospital
Rome, Italy

Robert Wade
Consultant Clinical Oncologist
Norfolk and Norwich University
Hospital
Norwich, UK

Cambridge, UK

Michael Williams
Consultant Clinical Oncologist
Cambridge University Hospitals NHS
Trust
Cambridge, UK

Glossary

Performance status (PS) The scales and criteria used to assess how the cancer affects the daily living abilities of patients and to determine appropriateness of treatment. The WHO/Eastern Cooperative Oncology Group (ECOG) PS used in this book is as follows:

0: fully active, no restrictions on activities

1: unable to do strenuous activities, but able to carry out light housework and sedentary activities

2: able to walk and manage self-care, but unable to work; out of bed for more than 50% of waking hours

3: confined to bed or a chair for more than 50% of waking hours; capable of limited self-care

4: completely disabled; totally confined to a bed or chair; unable to do any self-care

5: dead.

Staging Staging is done to assess the extent of disease, choose the appropriate treatment, and assess the likely outcome of the disease. TNM staging denotes tumour, node, and metastatic status. Composite staging involves grouping various T, N, and M combinations into four stages (I–IV). The following prefixes are added to staging to indicate the method of staging:

c: clinical staging based on physical examination, imaging and endoscopy

p: pathological staging after surgery

y: denotes staging after neoadjuvant therapy.

Neoadjuvant therapy Therapy is given *before* a definitive treatment such as surgery to facilitate the procedure and/or improve the chances of cure.

Adjuvant therapy Therapy is given *after* a definitive treatment such as surgery or radiotherapy with the aim of destroying micrometastatic residual disease and thereby increasing the chances of cure.

RECIST criteria (Response Evaluation Criteria in Solid Tumours) Criteria used to assess treatment effectiveness. Most often the assessment is made radiologically. Based on these criteria, treatment responses are categorized as complete response, partial response, stable disease, or progressive disease.

Gross tumour volume (GTV) The gross demonstrable extent and location of the tumour. The GTV is delineated using clinical (e.g. physical examination), anatomical (e.g. CT, MRI), and/or functional-imaging modalities (e.g. PET, functional MRI). In case of post-operative radiotherapy after complete macroscopic resection, there is no GTV to define and only a CTV needs to be delineated.

Clinical target volume (CTV) The volume of tissue that contains a demonstrable GTV and/or subclinical malignant disease with a certain probability of occurrence considered relevant for therapy. The definition of the CTV is derived from the extent of microscopic spread based on histological examination of post mortem or surgical specimens, biological characteristics of the tumour, local recurrence patterns, and the experience of the radiation oncologists.

Planning target volume (PTV) A geometrical concept introduced to ensure that the prescribed radiation dose will actually be delivered to all parts of the CTV with a clinically acceptable probability, despite geometrical uncertainties such as organ motion and setup variations. The PTV is derived by adding a margin to the CTV which takes into account the physiological organ motions and variations in patient positioning setup and alignment of the therapeutic beams during the treatment planning, and through all treatment sessions.

Atypical resection of liver A method of resection where the tumour is peeled out of liver parenchyma using a modern ultrasound knife. This allows the parenchyma to be crushed while leaving the bile ducts and vessels intact. Using this technique complete tumour removal can be performed regardless of the surgical resectability as defined by the anatomical borders of the liver segments.

ECOG - http://ecog.dfci.harvard.edu/general/perf_stat.html

TNM - http://www.uicc.org/resources/tnm

Case 1

Squamous cell carcinoma of unknown head and neck primary site

Suat W. Loo and Tom Roques

Case history

A 73-year-old white man presented with a 3-month history of right neck swelling. He had no other associated symptoms. He had never smoked and consumed alcohol only occasionally. His past medical history included hypertension and diet-controlled diabetes mellitus. His Eastern Cooperative Oncology Group (ECOG) performance status was 0. On clinical examination, there was a palpable right-sided level II lymph node. Flexible nasoendoscopy failed to identify a primary mucosal lesion. An ultrasound-guided core biopsy of the right neck node revealed poorly differentiated squamous cell carcinoma showing strong immunohistochemical staining for p16. Magnetic resonance imaging (MRI) demonstrated two necrotic lymph nodes in the right level II neck measuring 2.5 and 1.5cm in maximum dimension, respectively. Again, no definite primary site could be seen.

Questions

1. What investigation should be performed next?
2. What is the clinical and prognostic significance of p16 expression in tumour cells?

Answers

1. What investigation should be performed next?

Approximately 3% of patients with squamous cell carcinoma of the head and neck present with cervical lymph node metastasis from an unknown primary site. The most commonly affected nodal region is level II, and the majority present with N2a/b disease with unilateral lymph node involvement. Initial evaluation should include a detailed history, complete physical examination of the head and neck, flexible nasoendoscopy, imaging studies such as MRI of the head and neck, and needle biopsy of the cervical lymph node. If the primary tumour remains unidentified, a fluorine-18 fluorodeoxyglucose positron emission tomography–computed tomography (^{18}FDG PET-CT) scan should be performed next. This permits detection of occult primary tumours in up to 40% of patients. Lesions of the tonsil and base of the tongue are the primary tumours most commonly identified. It also allows identification of unsuspected metastases in the neck and distant sites.

2. What is the clinical and prognostic significance of p16 expression in tumour cells?

In 2007, the International Agency for Research on Cancer (IARC) convened a panel of experts to review data on the relationship between human papillomavirus (HPV) and squamous cell carcinoma of the head and neck. They concluded that HPV is a causative agent in oropharyngeal cancer. HPV-associated cancers most commonly arise from the tonsils of patients without the traditional risk factors of smoking and alcohol consumption. They usually present with early T stage and advanced N stage disease. Thus, HPV-associated oropharyngeal cancers are more likely to present as occult primary tumours. p16 positivity is commonly used as a surrogate marker of HPV status and is thus useful in the evaluation of patients presenting with squamous cell carcinoma with unknown head and neck primary site. The primary cancer is more likely to be located within the oropharynx if immunohistochemical analysis of tumour cells from the cervical nodes shows strong p16 expression. Similarly, the presence of Epstein–Barr virus in the cervical nodes suggests a nasopharyngeal primary tumour. p16-positive oropharyngeal cancers have a better prognosis than their p16-negative counterparts, with an estimated 50% reduction in the risk of death regardless of treatment modality.

The patient underwent PET-CT scanning. The scan results showed focal increased uptake of FDG in the right level II neck node with a maximum standardized uptake value of 8.3, corresponding to the two necrotic enlarged cervical nodes. No other lesions were seen.

Question

3. What further investigation should be performed?

Answer

3. What further investigation should be performed?

An evaluation under general anaesthesia (EUA) is the next step in the diagnostic workup of this patient. Obtaining PET-CT images prior to EUA has several advantages. It facilitates the evaluation and biopsy of suspicious areas of increased ^{18}FDG uptake and minimizes false positive results at biopsy sites which can be a problem if EUA preceded PET-CT. At EUA, all suspicious-looking lesions should be biopsied. Tonsillectomy and blind biopsies from the base of tongue, nasopharynx, and pyriform sinus should also be performed. This permits the detection of primary tumours that are too small to be visualized on PET-CT in up to 15% of cases. Approximately 80% of these lesions are located in the tonsil and tongue base.

An EUA was performed in this patient. Careful evaluation of the mucosal sites did not reveal any abnormalities. Bilateral tonsillectomy was carried out and blind biopsies were taken from the tongue base, post-nasal space, and pyriform sinus on both sides. No malignancy was found on histology.

Question

4. What is the optimal management of this patient?

Answer

4. What is the optimal management of this patient?

Due to a lack of randomized clinical studies, the optimal management of patients presenting with squamous cell carcinoma from an unknown head and neck primary site remains undefined. Treatment depends largely on the nodal stage at presentation. The priority is to achieve long-term loco-regional disease control. The risk of subsequent distant failure is considered low. Patients with N1 disease can be managed with single-modality treatment—either neck dissection or radiotherapy. Both options are equally effective and result in comparable nodal control rates. Post-operative radiotherapy is only indicated in those with extracapsular nodal extension and pathological N2 disease. Those with inoperable neck disease should be managed with radiotherapy and concurrent chemotherapy. In patients with N2 or N3 disease, irradiation of the bilateral neck and putative mucosal sites results in a reduction in the risk of subsequent loco-regional recurrence of tumour. As the majority of squamous cell carcinomas of unknown head and neck primaries are likely to have originated from the oropharynx, the base of the tongue and ipsilateral tonsil should be included within the clinical target volume (CTV). It is reasonable not to include the supraglottic or glottic larynx in the radiotherapy treatment volume. This is because damage to these structures, as well as the nearby pharyngeal constrictor muscles, by radiotherapy can result in long-term dysphagia and the risk of aspiration, with an adverse impact on the patient's quality of life. Nonetheless, it remains unclear whether irradiation of the bilateral neck and putative mucosal sites improves survival compared with the more limited approach of surgery and ipsilateral radiotherapy. Published results from single-centre series show excellent loco-regional control rates with acceptable long-term treatment-related complications with either approach. The primary mucosal tumour will subsequently emerge in approximately 25% of patients managed with neck dissection and adjuvant ipsilateral radiotherapy. Regular clinical follow-up after completion of treatment is therefore needed to look for recurrence of tumour or development of a second primary head and neck malignancy and to manage treatment-related complications.

The patient underwent irradiation of the bilateral neck and putative mucosal sites using intensity-modulated radiotherapy to a dose of 65Gy in 30 fractions over 6 weeks with concurrent weekly cisplatin. There was complete regression of the right level II cervical nodes and clinical evaluation 6 weeks post-treatment showed no residual disease.

Question

5. Does the patient require a post-treatment neck dissection?

Answer

5. Does the patient require a post-treatment neck dissection?

There has been debate over the role of planned neck dissection following chemo-radiotherapy in patients with N2 head and neck squamous cell carcinoma. Some clinicians recommend adjuvant neck dissection for all patients with N2 tumours regardless of treatment response, while others advocate its use only in those with residual nodal disease following chemoradiotherapy. There is now strong evidence to support the use of PET-CT in the evaluation of treatment response after chemo-radiotherapy. Patients with a negative PET-CT 3 months after completion of treatment can avoid neck dissection without the risk of regional recurrence. The negative predictive value of post-treatment PET-CT in this setting is greater than 95%.

Follow-up details of the case

PET-CT performed 3 months following chemoradiotherapy showed a complete metabolic and radiological response. The patient was observed. He was last reviewed at 32 months following treatment with no evidence of tumour recurrence and no late sequelae of treatment.

Further reading

Jereczek-Fossa BA, Jassem J, Orecchia R. Cervical lymph node metastases of squamous cell carcinoma from an unknown primary. *Cancer Treatment Reviews* 2004; **30**: 153–164.

Loo SW, Geropantas K, Beadsmoore C, et al. Neck dissection can be avoided after sequential chemoradiotherapy and negative post-treatment positron emission tomography-computed tomography in N2 head and neck squamous cell carcinoma. *Clinical Oncology (Royal College of Radiologists)* 2011; **23**: 512–517.

Lu H, Yao M, Tan H. Unknown primary head and neck cancer treated with intensity-modulated radiation therapy: to what extent the volume should be irradiated. *Oral Oncology* 2009; **45**: 474–479.

Waltonen JD, Ozer E, Hall NC, Schuller DE, Agrawal A. Metastatic carcinoma of the neck of unknown primary origin: evolution and efficacy of the modern workup. *Archives of Otolaryngology–Head and Neck Surgery* 2009; **135**: 1024–1029.

Case 2

Nasopharyngeal carcinoma

Suat W. Loo and Tom Roques

Case history

A 60-year-old white man presented with a 6-week history of epistaxis, nasal obstruction, headache, diplopia, and left neck swelling. On clinical examination, there was left-sided sixth cranial nerve palsy and a palpable cervical node in the left level II neck measuring 4cm in maximum dimension. Flexible nasoendoscopy showed a mass in the left nasopharynx. Biopsy confirmed a moderately differentiated non-keratinizing carcinoma. MRI revealed a soft tissue mass centred on the left nasopharynx with extension into the oropharynx and ipsilateral parapharyngeal space. There was marrow infiltration of the skull base with involvement of the left cavernous sinus (Fig. 2.1). Enlarged bilateral level II cervical nodes were present, the largest measuring 4.5cm in its greatest dimension. Computed tomography showed erosion of the skull base with no evidence of distant metastatic disease.

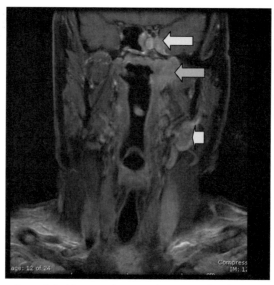

Fig. 2.1 MRI scan shows left side nasopharyngeal cancer with left cavernous sinus and paraoesophageal invasion, and enlarged upper deep cervical nodes

Questions

1. What is the histological classification of this patient's nasopharyngeal carcinoma according to the World Health Organization (WHO)?
2. What is the stage of this patient's nasopharyngeal carcinoma?
3. What is the optimal management?

Answers

1. What is the histological classification of this patient's nasopharyngeal carcinoma according to the World Health Organization (WHO)?

The WHO grading system divides nasopharyngeal carcinoma into keratinizing squamous cell carcinoma (WHO type I) and non-keratinizing carcinoma. The latter is in turn subdivided into differentiated (WHO type II) and undifferentiated carcinomas (WHO type III). Lymphoepithelioma is a WHO type III nasopharyngeal carcinoma characterized by a lymphoid infiltrate. Thus, this patient has a WHO type II nasopharyngeal carcinoma. Approximately 95% of affected patients from southern China have either WHO type II or III nasopharyngeal carcinoma whereas a quarter of those from the United States have WHO type I disease. The Epstein–Barr virus is associated with type II and III tumours. Undifferentiated nasopharyngeal carcinomas respond better to radiotherapy than differentiated ones; however, they have a higher rate of distant metastasis compared with their differentiated counterparts.

2. What is the stage of this patient's nasopharyngeal carcinoma?

There are two major staging systems in use for nasopharyngeal carcinoma: the 1997 revised American Joint Committee on Cancer (AJCC) TNM system (Fleming et al. 1997) and the Ho system (Ho 1978). The AJCC system is preferred in Europe and the United States. According to the AJCC TNM classification, this patient has T4N2M0 or stage IVA disease in view of the intracranial disease extension and the presence of bilateral involved cervical nodes less than 6cm in size. The majority of patients with nasopharyngeal carcinoma present with either stage III or IV disease.

3. What is the optimal management?

Radiotherapy to a curative dose is the cornerstone of management in nasopharyngeal carcinoma. The Intergroup 0099 Phase III Study (Al-Sarraf et al. 1998) showed improved survival with the addition of chemotherapy to radiotherapy in advanced-stage disease. In this study, patients with advanced-stage nasopharyngeal carcinoma were randomly assigned to receive either radiotherapy alone to 70Gy or the same radiotherapy schedule with three cycles of concurrent cisplatin followed by three cycles of adjuvant cisplatin and 5-fluorouracil (5-FU) chemotherapy. There was a statistically significant improvement in the 3-year survival rate from 47% to 78% with the addition of chemotherapy to radiotherapy. Based on the results of this study, the optimal management of this patient should be radiotherapy to a curative dose with concurrent platinum-based chemotherapy. The addition of induction chemotherapy is preferred, as the toxicities of concurrent chemoradiotherapy may preclude delivery of adjuvant chemotherapy. This treatment paradigm results in local tumour control rates of approximately 50–70% in T4 tumours and regional control rates of 70% in N2 disease. Neck dissection is reserved for those with persistent nodal disease following chemoradiotherapy. Although chemoradiotherapy is effective in nasopharyngeal carcinoma, it can also result in long-term treatment-related toxicities due to close proximity of the tumour to adjacent organs such as the major salivary glands, pituitary gland, temporal lobes, and the middle and inner ear. Xerostomia is one of the major late complications of chemoradiotherapy for nasopharyngeal carcinoma due to the high radiation doses received by the parotid glands. Consequently, techniques such as intensity-modulated radiotherapy have been explored in an attempt to improve the therapeutic ratio. By producing highly conformal dose distributions around the tumour volume with sparing of the adjacent uninvolved organs, intensity-modulated radiotherapy has the potential to reduce the long-term toxicity of treatment. Indeed, there is now randomized evidence to show that intensity-modulated radiotherapy reduces the incidence of severe late xerostomia compared with two-dimensional non-conformal techniques in patients with nasopharyngeal carcinoma treated with high-dose radiotherapy.

The patient was treated with three cycles of induction cisplatin and 5-FU chemotherapy followed by intensity-modulated radiotherapy to a dose of 66Gy in 33 fractions over 6.5 weeks with concurrent weekly carboplatin, achieving a complete response. Post-treatment MRI showed no evidence of persistent disease. Endoscopy and biopsies confirmed the absence of residual tumour. Four years following completion of treatment the patient re-presented with nasal obstruction and trismus. Flexible nasoendoscopy showed a lesion in the post-nasal space. Repeat imaging revealed local recurrence of tumour within the left nasopharynx with involvement of the ipsilateral medial ptyergoid muscle and skull base. Biopsies demonstrated recurrent nasopharyngeal carcinoma. [18]FDG PET-CT scan showed tracer uptake in the left nasopharynx with anterior extension into the pterygoid region with no evidence of nodal relapse or distant metastasis. His ECOG performance status remained 0 and he had no residual toxicity from his previous chemoradiotherapy.

Question

4. What is the optimal management of this patient's recurrent disease?

Answer

4. What is the optimal management of this patient's recurrent disease?

Despite the effectiveness of chemoradiotherapy, a significant proportion of patients with advanced-stage nasopharyngeal carcinoma will develop local recurrence of tumour. These patients have a poor prognosis if left untreated. Early stage local recurrences can be managed with salvage nasopharyngectomy, intracavity brachytherapy, or interstitial implants. Unfortunately more than half of all local recurrences present as rT3 or rT4 tumours. In these cases, surgery or brachytherapy are of limited benefit. Re-irradiation with external beam radiotherapy represents the only potentially curative treatment option (Fig. 2.2). However, it is associated with a significant risk of damage to normal tissue due to the close proximity of the recurrent tumour to adjacent critical organs. Several factors therefore need to be taken into consideration when considering re-irradiation for this group of patients. These include the time interval from the initial radiotherapy treatment, the radiation dose already delivered to the adjacent critical structures, the severity of existing late complications from previous radiotherapy, and the ECOG performance status of the patient. The risk of long-term treatment-related complications should be carefully discussed and appropriate consent obtained. During re-irradiation, the radiation dose to the adjacent critical structures should be kept as low as possible. This is best achieved using highly conformal techniques such as intensity-modulated radiotherapy. Available data from the published literature suggest that the toxicity from re-irradiating locally recurrent nasopharyngeal carcinoma is acceptable. In a patient series reported by Qiu et al. (2012), moderate to severe late toxicity was noted in 35.7% of patients treated with re-irradiation using intensity-modulated radiotherapy. Of these, 15.7% had posterior nasal space ulceration, 24.3% experienced cranial nerve palsy, 17.1% developed trismus, and

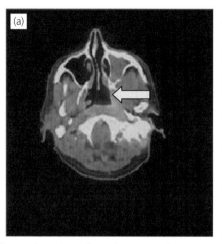
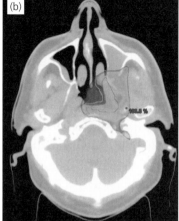

Fig. 2.2 (See also colour plate section)

17.1% experienced deafness. There are now an increasing number of published single-institution reports on the use of intensity-modulated radiotherapy in the re-irradiation of radio-recurrent nasopharyngeal carcinoma showing promising survival outcomes. With careful patient selection, 5-year survival rates of up to 42% for rT3 and 17% for rT4 tumours can be achieved. As a result, re-irradiation is now considered to be standard practice in the management of radio-recurrent nasopharyngeal carcinoma. The patient in this case study has locally advanced recurrent nasopharyngeal carcinoma with extension into the masticator space and skull base. He is thus unsuitable for salvage surgery or brachytherapy. Despite his recurrent disease, his ECOG performance status remains excellent. Moreover, it is 4 years since his initial radiotherapy and he has no residual toxicity from his previous treatment. The optimal management is thus re-irradiation with intensity-modulated radiotherapy.

Treatment details and outcome of the case

The patient was re-irradiated using intensity-modulated radiotherapy to a dose of 60Gy in 30 fractions with concurrent weekly cisplatin. He tolerated treatment well with minimal acute toxicity. Unfortunately, he died of persistent local disease 4 months following completion of treatment.

Further reading

Al-Sarraf M, Leblanc M, Giri S, et al. Chemoradiotherapy versus radiotherapy in patients with advanced nasopharyngeal cancer: phase III randomized Intergroup Study 0099. *Journal of Clinical Oncology* 1998; **16**: 1310–1317.

Chang JT, See LC, Liao CT, et al. Locally recurrent nasopharyngeal carcinoma. *Radiotherapy and Oncology* 2000; **54**: 135–142.

Fleming ID, Cooper JS, Henson DE, et al. (eds) *AJCC cancer staging manual*, 5th edn. Philadelphia: Lippincott-Raven, 1997; 33–35.

Ho JH. Stage classification of nasopharyngeal carcinoma: a review. In: *Nasopharyngeal carcinoma: etiology and control*, IARC Scientific Publication No. 20, 1978; 99–113.

Pow EH, Kwong DL, McMillan AS, et al. Xerostomia and quality of life after intensity-modulated radiotherapy vs. conventional radiotherapy for early-stage nasopharyngeal carcinoma: initial report on a randomized controlled clinical trial. *International Journal of Radiation Oncology Biology Physics* 2006; **66**: 981–991.

Qiu S, Lin S, Tham IW, Pan J, Lu J, Lu JJ. Intensity-modulated radiation therapy in the salvage of locally recurrent nasopharyngeal carcinoma. *International Journal of Radiation Oncology Biology Physics* 2012; **83**: 676–683.

Shanmugaratnam K, Sobin LH. Histological typing of tumors of upper respiratory tract and ear. In: *International histological classification of tumours*, 2nd edn (ed. Shanmugaratnam K, Sobin LH). Geneva: WHO, 1991; 32–33.

Case 3

Small cell lung cancer during pregnancy

Thankamma Ajithkumar

Case history

A 37-year-old woman presented with pneumonia for which she received intravenous antibiotics. Six months later she re-presented with left-sided chest discomfort and increasing breathlessness. She was 21 weeks pregnant. She was afebrile, and her blood tests were unremarkable. She had a chest X-ray (Fig. 3.1).

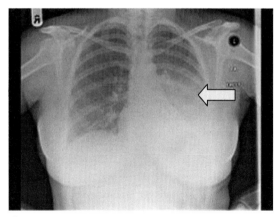

Fig. 3.1

Questions

1. What does the chest X-ray show and what are the differential diagnoses?
2. How will you investigate further?

Answers

1. What does the chest X-ray show and what are the differential diagnoses?

The chest X-ray shows a haziness of the left lower zone with a possible left hilar shadow and obliteration of the left costophrenic angle. The differential diagnoses include infection, pleural effusion, interstitial lung disease, pulmonary embolism, drug-induced lung abnormalities, and malignancy.

2. How will you investigate further?

Cancer during pregnancy poses a challenging situation in terms of providing optimal care to the woman without harming the foetus. Radiological investigations should be undertaken only if absolutely necessary and foetal exposure to ionizing radiation should be kept to a safe level. Foetal radiation exposure at a dose of 1mGy is considered to be safe, but foetal exposure at doses of >1–2cGy should especially be avoided during the first trimester (organogenesis) and the second trimester (continuing development of brain, teeth, and eyes) (see Table 3.1). Chest X-ray, ultrasound examination, upper gastrointestinal (GI) endoscopy, bronchoscopy, lumbar puncture, and bone marrow examination are safe. MRI is safe and can be useful for ruling out brain and liver metastases, though gadolinium should be avoided during the first trimester. Abdominal–pelvic CT and radio-isotope scans should be avoided. However, CT scans are not absolutely contraindicated in pregnancy. They can be performed if there is a safe distance between the radiation field and the uterus such as to keep foetal radiation exposure to below 1cGy (e.g. head and neck, extremities, and a limited area of chest) (Table 3.2). A bronchoscopic evaluation and ultrasound scan of the abdomen to rule out liver metastasis are safe. If a radiological physicist is available to calculate the foetal radiation dose, the woman can have a limited CT scan of the chest.

Table 3.1 Radiation dose to uterus/foetus during various radiological investigations

Investigation	Uterine/foetal dose (Gy)
Chest X-ray	0.000005
Abdominal X-ray	0.022
Mammogram	0.04
Chest CT scan	0.002
Abdominal CT scan	0.02
Pelvic CT scan	0.07
Barium enema	0.036
Intravenous urogram	0.045
Bone scan	0.018–0.455

Table 3.2 Foetal radiation dose during radical radiotherapy of various tumour sites

Tumour site	Foetal radiation dose (Gy)
Cervix	45–50
Mantle field for lymphoma	0.014–0.13
Breast	0.14–0.18
Brain and head and neck	0.0015–0.08

She had a limited CT scan of the chest with abdominal shielding (Fig. 3.2).

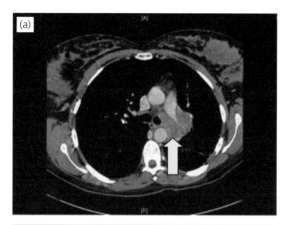

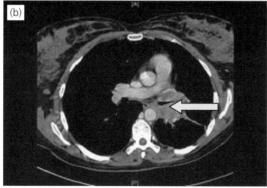

Fig. 3.2

Question

3. What does the CT scan show?

Answer

3. What does the CT scan show?

The CT scan shows a bulky mediastinal lymphadenopathy, predominantly on the left side (3.2A) associated with a mass in the left lower lobe of the lung surrounding the left main bronchus, causing narrowing of the lumen (3.2B). There is also associated thickening of the horizontal fissure. No pleural effusion or bone disease is evident on the available scans.

The radiological appearances of different subtypes of lung cancer vary. Small cell lung cancer typically presents as large central masses with atelectasis and extensive mediastinal lymphadenopathy. Squamous cell carcinoma presents as a large central tumour with atelectasis and mediastinal lymphadenopathy. Adenocarcinoma presents as small peripheral lesions with a high propensity for nodal and distant spread. Large cell carcinoma presents as large peripheral lesions with a high propensity for regional lymph nodes and distant metastasis.

Bronchoscopic biopsy showed small cell lung cancer, and abdominal ultrasound did not show any liver metastasis.

Questions

4. What are the challenges in the management of this woman?
5. Outline your management.

Answers

4. What are the challenges in the management of this woman?

From the available information, this woman, who is more than 21 weeks' pregnant, has a limited stage small cell lung cancer. Small cell lung cancer grows rapidly and the median survival is 2–4 months without treatment. The standard management is concurrent chemoradiotherapy followed by prophylactic cranial irradiation (PCI), which results in a median survival of 15–20 months with 20–40% surviving to 2 years. Her pregnancy is well into second trimester, which makes a medical termination risky. Thus, she needs urgent treatment while continuing pregnancy.

Most chemotherapy drugs have a molecular weight of <600kDa, and therefore can cross the placenta. Chemotherapy during the first trimester is associated with a 17–25% risk of malformations or foetal death and hence is best avoided. Chemotherapy may be given relatively safely during the second or third trimester, with a 5–7% incidence of intrauterine growth retardation, a 5% incidence of still birth, a 5% incidence of premature delivery, a 4% incidence of bone narrow suppression, and a 3–5% incidence of foetal death. There are no data on the safety of new targeted agents.

5. Outline your management.

Radiotherapy is contraindicated at this stage. The best option is to treat her with chemotherapy until elective delivery of the foetus. The standard chemotherapy regimen for small cell lung cancer is cisplatin/etoposide. Cisplatin has been used safely during pregnancy to treat non-small cell lung cancer, ovarian cancer, and cervical cancer at a dose similar to the standard dose in a non-pregnant woman. However, there are limited data on the safety of etoposide in pregnancy.

A multidisciplinary approach, including input from gynaecologists and neonatologists, is needed to coordinate care of the woman and her foetus. The patient can be treated with chemotherapy until 3 weeks prior to elective delivery.

A recommendation to start a combination of cisplatin/etoposide at the non-pregnant standard dose for four courses followed by elective delivery of the foetus was made.

A chest X-ray after four courses of chemotherapy showed complete resolution of the previously noted left lung shadow. Subsequently she had an elective caesarean section and a healthy baby girl was delivered.

Questions

6. What are the important aspects of delivery and post-partum management?
7. What would be your further management of small cell lung cancer?

Answers

6. What are the important aspects of delivery and post-partum management?

Elective delivery is generally planned after 32–35 weeks' gestation (earlier in modern neonatal units which have a better outcome for babies) and 3 weeks after the last chemotherapy to allow for full bone marrow recovery of the woman and foetus and for placental drug excretion from the foetus. Since there is a risk of placental metastasis, the placenta should be sent for histopathological examination. The baby needs a full clinical examination for any obvious metastasis. Breast feeding is not recommended during and up to 2–4 weeks after completion of systemic cancer treatment. With platinum-based chemotherapy during pregnancy, there is a concern that any non-renally excreted drug will be retained within the tissue which may affect later development of the child (e.g. neural), although there is little evidence of this. The optimal follow-up of a healthy baby is not known.

7. What would be your further management of small cell lung cancer?

Following delivery, this woman needs re-staging, including a CT scan of the brain, chest, abdomen, and pelvis followed by further treatment. Patients with limited stage small cell lung cancer are treated with chemotherapy along with concurrent radiotherapy, which improves 3-year survival by 5.4%. Patients generally receive four to six courses of platinum-based chemotherapy. Meta-analyses show that early radiotherapy improves long-term survival, and a short time between the first day of chemotherapy and the last day of thoracic radiotherapy is also associated with improved survival. However, there is no evidence to recommend concurrent chemoradiotherapy at this stage, though it is an option. In the absence of progressive disease after initial treatment, PCI is also recommended. This improves 3-year survival by 6% and results in a better disease-free survival and lower cumulative incidence of subsequent brain metastases.

Restaging did not show any evidence of residual disease. She subsequently received radiotherapy to the chest concurrent with the fifth course of chemotherapy, and after six courses of chemotherapy she underwent PCI.

Five months after the completion of PCI, she presented with persistent vomiting for 2 weeks. She denied any headache, convulsions, or chest symptoms. Her ECOG performance status was 0. Clinical examination and CT staging (including of the brain) was normal. She underwent a gadolinium-enhanced MRI scan (Fig. 3.3).

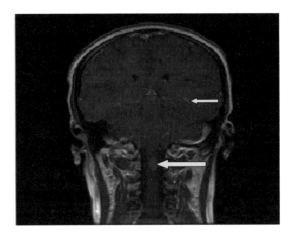

Fig. 3.3

Questions

8. What does the MRI show?
9. How will you manage her?

Answers

8. What does the MRI show?

MRI shows irregular leptomeningeal enhancement. There is also an irregular contrast-enhancing intramedullary lesion in the cervical spinal cord. This appearance is suggestive of leptomeningeal carcinomatosis.

9. How will you manage her?

She needs restaging with CT scan of the chest and abdomen and examination of the cerebrospinal fluid (CSF). CSF examination will show increased opening pressure, increased leukocytes, elevated protein, and decreased glucose. Malignant cells may be seen in >80% of cases. If malignant cells are seen in the CSF, repeat CSF examination will be useful to assess response to and to guide intrathecal treatment.

Since she has radiological evidence of leptomeningeal disease with a threatening lesion in the cervical cord and is of ECOG performance status 0, she would benefit from urgent radiotherapy to the spinal cord, to prevent any potential neurological morbidity (20–30Gy in five to ten fractions), and from intrathecal chemotherapy.

The median survival of untreated patients with leptomeningeal disease is 4–6 weeks. Radiotherapy is useful for relieving symptoms caused by tumour bulk or for ventricular outflow obstruction. Intrathecal chemotherapy increases the median survival to 4–6 months in candidates who are a 'good risk' (see Fig. 3.4), with a 1-year survival of 15%. Intrathecal drug administration using an intraventricular reservoir system (Ommaya reservoir) results in a uniform distribution and consistent levels of drug in the CSF space. It is more tolerable for patients and safer than repeated lumbar punctures. The benefit of systemic chemotherapy in the absence of systemic disease is not known.

Progress and follow-up of this case

This patient received intrathecal methotrexate (Fig. 3.4) along with six courses of oral topotecan (second-line chemotherapy for small cell lung cancer). While on maintenance intrathecal methotrexate, she developed pneumonia and died 28 months after her initial diagnosis.

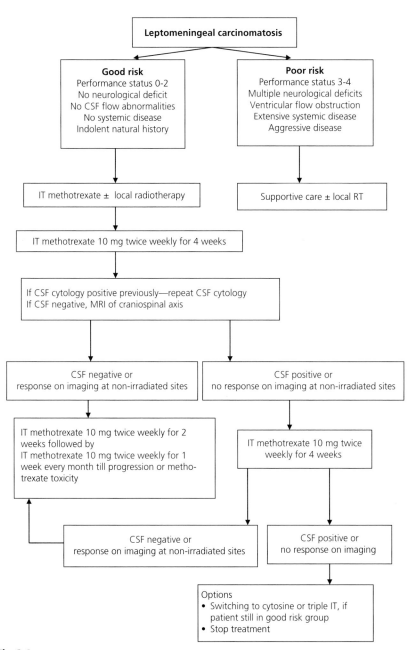

Fig. 3.4

Further reading

Azim Jr AA, Peccatorib FA, Pavlidis N. Lung cancer in the pregnant woman: to treat or not to treat, that is the question. *Lung Cancer* 2010; **67**: 251–256.

Chamberlain MC. Leptomeningeal metastasis. *Current Opinion in Oncology* 2010; **22**: 627–635.

Garridoa M, Claverob J, Huetec A, et al. Prolonged survival of a woman with lung cancer diagnosed and treated with chemotherapy during pregnancy. Review of cases reported. *Lung Cancer* 2008; **60**: 285–290.

van Meerbeeck JP, Fennell DA, De Ruysscher DKM. Small-cell lung cancer. *The Lancet* 2011; **378**: 1741–1755.

Rossi A, Martelli O, Di Maio M. Treatment of patients with small-cell lung cancer: from meta-analyses to clinical practice. *Cancer Treatment Reviews* 2012; **39**: 498–506.

Case 4

Breast metastasis from non-small cell lung cancer

Thankamma Ajithkumar

Case history

A 60-year-old woman presented with a 4-week history of mass in the right breast. A screening mammogram 6 months before had shown no evidence of any mass lesion. Her mother had had breast cancer at the age of 60. A mammogram showed a suspicious lesion in the upper outer quadrant of right breast. An ultrasound confirmed a superficial 1.3cm irregular mass with no associated axillary lymphadenopathy. Biopsy of the breast mass showed a carcinoma of ductal origin, which was negative for oestrogen (ER), progesterone (PgR), and gross cystic disease fluid protein-15 (GCDFP-15), and positive for thyroid transcription factor 1 (TTF-1).

Questions

1. What is the pathological diagnosis?
2. How will you proceed?

Answers

1. What is the pathological diagnosis?

The negative immunohistochemistry for ER, PgR, and GCDFP-15 suggests that it is a metastasis to the breast rather than a primary breast cancer. Although ER/PgR negativity does not rule out a primary breast cancer, GCDFP-15 helps to identify metastatic breast cancer in the absence of a previous history of breast cancer and/or in tumours which are negative for ER and PgR. A positive GCDFP-15 suggests primary breast cancer of ductal origin but a negative result does not exclude it due to a low sensitivity of 60–75%.

TTF-1 is a tissue-specific transcription factor expressed in epithelial cells of the lung and the thyroid. Some 70–80% of primary lung adenocarcinomas express TTF-1. A literature review showed that only four out of 419 breast cancers expressed TTF-1 (Maounis et al. 2010). Therefore the most probable diagnosis is metastatic non-small cell lung cancer (NSCLC).

2. How will you proceed?

This woman needs a chest X-ray and CT staging of the thorax, abdomen, and pelvis to look for a lung primary and to rule out further metastatic disease.

The chest X-ray and CT scan are shown in Fig. 4.1.

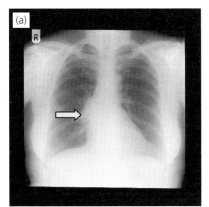 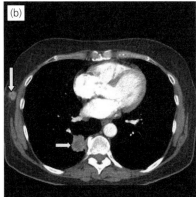

Fig. 4.1

Question

3. What do the images show?

Answer

3. What do the images show?

The chest X-ray shows a right hilar mass. Since the right heart border is well defined, the lesion will be arising posterior to the heart. The axial CT images show a stellate mass in the right breast (metastasis) and an irregular mass in the right lower lobe (primary tumour).

The scan also showed a 1.3cm right hilar node and 1.2cm subcarinal node (not shown in Fig. 4.1). There was no disease elsewhere.

Question

4. What is the further management?

Answer

4. What is the further management?

This patient has a radiological T2N2M1b lung cancer. It is important to establish the true extent of the metastatic disease, and there are at least two clinical scenarios with potentially different treatment approaches. These include:

1. Disseminated metastatic disease with involvement of mediastinal nodes and possibly other occult disease, when treatment is palliative with systemic chemotherapy.

2. Oligometastatic disease—the only sites of disease are in the lung and breast with the nodes being reactive. In this situation a more radical approach should be considered.

Therefore further investigations should include a PET scan, a biopsy from the lung lesion to confirm a lung primary and to correlate with the breast pathology, and epidermal growth factor receptor (EGFR) mutation status.

A PET scan showed intense fluorodeoxyglucose (FDG) uptake in the breast lump (SUV 11.5), lung mass (SUV 12), right hilar nodes (SUV 4.3), and subcarinal nodes (SUV 4.6) but without other uptake. Figure 4.2 shows FDG uptake in the breast lump, the lung mass, and hilar nodes.

A biopsy from the lung tumour showed a poorly differentiated adenocarcinoma with areas of necrosis. The tumour cells were strongly positive for TTF1 and negative for ER and GCDFP-15. EGFR mutation testing was not available at the time this patient was diagnosed.

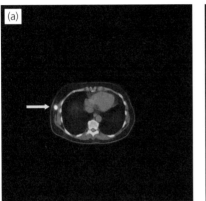 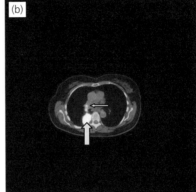

Fig. 4.2 (See also colour plate section)

Question

5. How will you proceed?

Answer

5. How will you proceed?

The features of the lung tumour correlate with those of the breast lump, suggesting the diagnosis of breast metastasis from adenocarcinoma of lung. The PET scan suggests possible involvement of the hilar and subcarinal nodes.

^{18}FDG PET/CT has an established role in the staging of NSCLC. It distinguishes malignant lung tumours from benign lesions more accurately than CT or PET alone.

PET/CT can detect malignant disease in normal-sized lymph nodes and therefore is more sensitive than CT scan alone. With regards to nodal staging, PET/CT has an equal or superior negative predictive value (i.e. the probability of not having the disease when the scan is negative) to mediastinoscopy. Therefore if lymph nodes are negative on PET/CT, a mediastinoscopy is not needed for confirmation. However, a PET scan has a poor positive predictive value with a high chance of false-positivity, leading incorrectly to upstaging of the disease. Thus, PET-positive regional nodes require histological confirmation to prove or refute metastasis.

PET/CT has a greater sensitivity than CT scan alone in detecting metastatic disease, except for brain and possibly liver metastases. Ideally, this woman should have a mediastinoscopy with histopathological examination of the PET-positive nodes to confirm or rule out nodal disease.

The multidisciplinary team decided not offer a mediastinoscopy, but recommended proceeding with four courses of chemotherapy with carboplatin and pemetrexed.

After four courses of chemotherapy CT restaging reported that the right lower lobe tumour had decreased in size from 3.4cm × 5.6cm to 2.6cm × 3.7cm with no change in the size of either the left hilar node or the subcarinal node. The breast metastasis decreased in size from 1.4cm × 1.3cm to 9mm × 11mm.

Questions

6. What is your further management?
7. Is there any role for surgery in this patient?

Answers

6. What is your further management?

In view of the decrease in size of the lung tumour and breast lump, with no change in the size of the nodes, it is reasonable to assume that the nodal disease is false positive on PET. Therefore the patient should be offered a mediastinoscopy to reassess the mediastinal nodes.

7. Is there any role for surgery in this patient?

Generally, patients with stage IV NSCLC have incurable disease. Patients with oligometastatic disease represent a distinct subset of patients with metastatic disease and a number of retrospective series have examined the role of surgical resection in patients with oligometastases. Following surgical resection of solitary brain metastases the 5-year survival is 11–30% and following adrenelectomy for solitary adrenal metastases the 5-year survival is 26%.

Reports of successful surgical resection in oligometastatic NSCLC at sites other than brain and adrenal are sparse. Breast metastasis (either synchronous or metachronous) from NSCLC is very unusual and patients have a poor prognosis, with most patients dying within in a year of diagnosis. Due to the rarity of the situation, there is no clear evidence to recommend surgery in this patient. Therefore any recommendation for an attempted surgical resection would be based on a perceived clinical benefit extrapolated from the literature on oligometastatic disease at other sites.

Mediastinocopy with samples from stations 4R and 7 did not show any evidence of malignancy. MRI of the brain was normal and CT staging did not show progression. She underwent a right lower lobectomy and excision of the solitary breast metastasis. Pathology showed ypT2aN0 R0 resection of lung and an Rx resection of the breast metastasis (due to a diathermized edge).

Fifteen months after surgery she presented with features suggestive of a stroke. CT and MRI of the brain showed a solitary left frontal lesion suggestive of a metastasis.

Questions

8. What is your management?
9. Should this patient have been offered PCI after surgery?

Answers

8. What is your management?

The patient needs to be started on high-dose steroids to minimize any cerebral oedema. Further staging with a CT scan of chest, abdomen, and pelvis is recommended to rule out systemic disease. Provided her ECOG performance status is good (0–1) and she has no systemic disease, she should be managed similarly to patients presenting with a single brain metastasis with surgery, radiotherapy, or a combination of both (see p. 54).

9. Should this patient have been offered PCI after surgery?

There is no proven role for PCI in NSCLC. Previous randomized trials have shown that although PCI decreases and/or delays brain metastases there is no survival benefit and there are concerns over long-term toxicity. These data have been confirmed by the report of the RTOG 0214 trial (Gore et al. 2011). Therefore this patient should not have been offered PCI.

Progress and follow-up

CT staging did not show any systemic disease, and hence the patient underwent complete resection of the single metastasis followed by whole-brain radiotherapy. She remains well without recurrent disease at 18 months follow-up, which is 3.5 years after her initial presentation.

Further reading

Gomez DR, Niibe Y, Chang JY. Oligometastatic disease at presentation or recurrence for nonsmall cell lung cancer. *Pulmonary Medicine* 2012; doi: 10.1155/2012/396592 [online only].

Gore EM, Bae K, Wong SJ, et al. Phase III comparison of prophylactic cranial irradiation versus observation in patients with locally advanced non-small-cell lung cancer: primary analysis of radiation therapy oncology group study RTOG 0214. *Clinical Oncology* 2011; 29: 272–278.

Ji FF, Gao P, Wang JG, et al. Contralateral breast metastasis from pulmonary adenocarcinoma: two case reports and literature review. *Thoracic Disease* 2012; 4: 384–389.

Maounis N, Chorti M, Legaki S et al. Metastasis to the breast from an adenocarcinoma of the lung with extensive micropapillary component: a case report and review of the literature. *Diagnostic Pathology* 2010; 5: 82 [online only].

Pfannschmidt J, Dienemann H. Surgical treatment of oligometastatic non-small cell lung cancer. *Lung Cancer*, 2010; 69: 251–258.

Case 5

Lung cancer in non-smokers

Spyridon Gennatas and Sanjay Popat

Case history

A 67-year-old South Asian woman who had never smoked presented with a 3-month history of back pain, dry cough, and increasing malaise. Her ECOG performance status was 2. A CT scan demonstrated a right upper lobe primary lung tumour, bilateral mediastinal and ipsilateral supraclavicular nodal involvement, bilateral lung metastases involving all lung lobes, and left adrenal and widespread bony metastases. Spinal MRI confirmed multiple vertebral metastases with threatened spinal cord compression at multiple levels. She received 20Gy in five fractions of radiotherapy to C7–T3 and T11–L1. Ultrasound-guided biopsy of an involved right supraclavicular fossa node confirmed adenocarcinoma positive for cytokeratin 7 (CK7), TTF-1, Napsin A, and carcinoembryonic antigen (CEA) and negative for cytokeratin 20 (CK20), caudal type homeobox 2 (CDX2), and GCDFP-15 by immunohistochemistry. These features were consistent with lung adenocarcinoma.

Questions

1. What is the stage of the patient's disease?
2. What other investigations need to be undertaken prior to deciding on a treatment plan?
3. What is the significance of a history of never smoking in patients with lung cancer?

Answers

1. What is the stage of the patient's disease?

T4 N3 M1b:

T4   – separate tumour nodule(s) within an ipsilateral lobe

N3   – contralateral mediastinal and ipsilateral supraclavicular lymph nodes

M1b – distant metastases (bone and adrenal).

2. What other investigations need to be undertaken prior to deciding on a treatment plan?

The tumour needs to be tested for *EGFR* mutations.

3. What is the significance of a history of never smoking in patients with lung cancer?

Lung cancer is generally associated with tobacco exposure. However, occurrence in patients who have never smoked is well recognized. In thoracic oncology, a 'never-smoker' has arbitrarily been defined as smoking 100 or fewer cigarettes over a lifetime. The WHO estimates that never-smokers account for 25% of new cases of lung cancer worldwide. Whether the incidence of never-smokers with lung cancer is increasing or whether a decrease in smoking-related lung cancers has been observed remains unclear, since tobacco exposure is poorly documented in most registries.

There is no conclusive evidence that mean age at presentation differs between never-smokers and smokers with lung cancer, although most studies indicate peak incidence is perhaps at a younger age in never-smokers. Lung cancer in never-smokers is wholly associated with adenocarcinoma (or variants thereof), whilst squamous carcinomas and small cell lung cancer are typically associated with tobacco. Indeed, pathological review is recommended in the case of such tumours diagnosed without tobacco exposure. A number of risk factors are recognized that are important not only in never-smokers but in smokers too. These include hereditary risks, exposure to environmental pollution—including second-hand tobacco smoke and cooking and heating fumes—and ionizing radiation. An increased incidence in women is observed, and this might reflect hormonal factors, with ER receptors expressed more commonly in lung cancer tissue than normal lung tissue and potentially correlating with poorer outcomes. Other risk factors include infections, particularly viral, low socio-economic status, immunosuppression, and diabetes mellitus.

Recently, a number of somatic molecular aberrations that are principally observed in never-smokers have been shown in a type of lung cancer that appears to be a distinct clinical entity—it is composed of different subtypes of carcinoma driven by different molecular aberrations. These will be discussed in more detail in the following sections.

EGFR mutation analysis was performed and a mutation was detected. This was an EGFR exon 19 deletion.

Questions

4. How common are *EGFR* mutations in lung cancer? Are there any particular subgroups more likely to harbour such mutations?

5. What *EGFR* mutations have been identified and which ones are associated with response to treatment with tyrosine kinase inhibitors (TKIs)?

6. Which TKIs are licensed for the first-line treatment of *EGFR*-mutant adenocarcinomas and what evidence supports their use?

7. What other molecular markers have been identified that could guide treatment decisions in lung cancer and what is their relationship to smoking status?

8. Are there any drugs that are currently licensed for any of these indications?

Answers

4. How common are *EGFR* mutations in lung cancer? Are there any particular subgroups more likely to harbour such mutations?

NSCLC can be divided into subgroups based solely on genetically discrete subsets according to the activating mutations they harbour. Somatic *EGFR* mutations were first identified in NSCLC in 2004 and were associated with a dramatic response to gefitinib. Since then considerable research has defined the relationship between genotype and clinical demographics. Mutations are more prevalent in East Asians, women, and never-smokers. They are predominantly observed in adenocarcinomas that tend to be TTF-1 positive. The exact prevalence of mutations is difficult to define since studies have used different denominators. However, prevalence varies by ethnicity, ranging from 5% in American current smokers, to 28% in American never-smokers, and as high as 68% in East Asian never-smokers. Prevalence seems to be inversely proportional to tobacco pack-years exposure.

5. What *EGFR* mutations have been identified and which ones are associated with response to treatment with tyrosine kinase inhibitors (TKIs)?

Activating *EGFR* mutations are restricted to exons 18–21 which encode the tyrosine kinase domain and result in constitutional activation of the kinase. Exon 19 mutations and the exon 21 L858R missense mutation account for about 90% of mutations. The remaining 10% are therefore rare, and are a mixture of missense, insertional, and deletional mutations.

Patients harbouring *EGFR* exon 19 deletions and L858R point mutations have impressively good outcomes from EGFR TKI-directed therapy. Exon 20 insertions are uncommon but are well recognized at presentation, and such tumours are typically resistant to EGFR TKI therapy.

6. Which TKIs are licensed for the first-line treatment of *EGFR*-mutant adenocarcinomas and what evidence supports their use?

In 2005 two trials first demonstrated the superiority of two EGFR TKIs (gefitinib and erlotinib) over placebo in certain patient subsets. The BR.21 phase III trial demonstrated that erlotinib prolonged survival in relapsed NSCLC following progression on first- or second-line chemotherapy compared with placebo (6.7 versus 4.7 months) (Shepherd et al. 2005). High response rates were observed in East Asian patients with the *EGFR* mutation who had never smoked. The ISEL phase III study investigating gefitinib in a similar population to the BR.21 trial did not show an overall survival advantage over placebo in the intention-to-treat population, but a benefit was identified in never-smokers and East Asian patients (Thatcher et al. 2005).

Since then, seven randomized phase III trials have since shown TKIs to be superior to platinum-doublet chemotherapy for progression-free survival (PFS), overall response rate (ORR), and quality of life in first-line patients with *EGFR* mutation. The first was the IPASS study, which compared gefitinib versus carboplatin and paclitaxel in never-smokers or ex-light smokers from East Asia with adenocarcinoma, a population enriched in patients with *EGFR* mutation. Despite this, only 59.7% of these adenocarcinomas harboured *EGFR* mutations, indicating that clinical demographics alone are inadequate in predicting somatic mutation and that molecular screening is required. In the subgroup with *EGFR* mutation a significantly increased PFS was seen with gefitinib [median 9.5 versus 6.3 months; hazard ratio (HR) 0.48 (95% confidence interval 0.36–0.64); *P* < 0.001]. The ORR favoured gefitinib (71.2 versus 47.3%), and underpinned significant improvements in quality of life domains in the gefitinib group. Similar outcomes were observed in the First-SIGNAL trial investigating a similar group of clinically selected Korean patients likely to have *EGFR* mutation. A benefit on overall survival (OS) was not observed in either trial due to post-progression crossover therapy.

Subsequently, four phase III trials have confirmed the superiority of gefitinib or erlotinib over platinum-doublet chemotherapy in first-line patients proven to

Table 5.1 Phase III Trials of gefitinib/erlotinib versus chemotherapy in first-line patients with *EGFR* mutant non-small-cell lung cancer

Trial and no. of patients	Setting	TKI	Comparator chemotherapy	Median PFS (months)	PFS HR (95% CI)	ORR (%)
1. Trials of clinically selected patients. *EGFR* mutation status included in subset analysis						
IPASS* (Mok et al. 2009) (*n* = 261)	East Asia	Gefitinib	Carboplatin– paclitaxel	9.5 vs 6.3, *P* < 0.001	0.48 (0.36–0.64)	71 vs 47
First-SIGNAL* (Lee et al. 2009) (*n* = 53)	Korea	Gefitinib	Cisplatin– gemcitabine	7.9 vs 2.1, *P* < 0.001	0.385 (0.208– 0.711)	55 vs 46
2. Trials of molecularly selected patients (*EGFR* L858R or exon 19 deletions only)						
NEJ002† (Maemondo et al. 2010) (*n* = 230)	East Asia	Gefitinib	Carboplatin– paclitaxel	10.8 vs 5.4, *P* < 0.001	0.30 (0.22–0.41)	73.7 vs 30.7
WJTOG3405† (Mitsudomi 2011) (*n* = 172)	East Asia	Gefitinib	Cisplatin– docetaxel	9.2 vs 6.3, *P* < 0.001	0.489 (0.336– 0.710)	62 vs 32
OPTIMAL† (Zhou et al. 2011) (*n* = 165)	China	Erlotinib	Carboplatin– gemcitabine	13.1 vs 4.6, *P* < 0.001	0.16 (0.10–0.26)	83 vs 36
EURTAC† (Rosell et al. 2012) (*n* = 174)	Europe	Erlotinib	Cisplatin/ carboplatin– docetaxel or gemcitabine	9.7 vs 5.2, *P* < 0.001	0.37 (0.25–0.54)	58 vs 15

CI, confidence interval; HR, hazard ratio; ORR; overall response rate; PFS, progression-free survival; TKI, tyrosine kinase inhibitor.
*Study population unselected for *EGFR* mutations. *n* is the number in the *EGFR* mutant subset.
†Study population selected for *EGFR* mutations.

harbour *EGFR* L858R or exon 19 deletions (Table 5.1), and as a result both are licensed for this indication. *EGFR* mutation testing should now therefore be performed on all patients eligible for TKI treatment and on mutation-positive patients treated with first-line EGFR TKI.

Acquired resistance to EGFR TKI has been shown to be mediated in about 40% of patients through a second *EGFR* mutation, T790M (exon 20). Such resistance can be overcome *in vitro* by irreversible EGFR inhibitors, which specifically inhibit T790M (e.g. afatinib or dacomitinib) and therefore have the potential to delay acquired resistance.

Afatinib (BIBW2992) is one such pan-ErbB-family (EGFR, HER2, ErbB3, and ErbB4) TKI, and has a proven advantage for PFS over placebo in relapsed *EGFR*-mutant NSCLC with acquired gefitinib/erlotinib resistance. Most recently, first-line afatinib has been shown to be superior to cisplatin–pemetrexed in patients with *EGFR* mutant adenocarcinoma [median PFS 13.61 versus 6.9 months for L858R/exon 19 deletion; HR 0.58 (0.43–0.78), $P = 0.0004$; objective response rate 56 versus 23%, $P < 0.0001$]. However, toxicities were frequent (afatinib toxicity, grade 3/4 diarrhoea in 14.4%).

7. What other molecular markers have been identified that could guide treatment decisions in lung cancer and what is their relationship to smoking status?

(a) Anaplastic lymphoma kinase (*ALK*).

In 2007 *ALK-EML4* gene rearrangements were identified in NSCLC. Since then a number of rarer non-*ALK* fusion partners have been identified. *ALK* rearrangements can be identified by a number of methods including fluorescence *in situ* hybridization (FISH), reverse transcriptase polymerase chain reaction, and immunohistochemistry, since the fusion protein is not normally expressed. *ALK* rearrangements are primarily identified in adenocarcinomas and are uncommon (with a prevalence of 2.4–5.6%). They are more frequent in younger patients (median 50 years) and never-smokers or light smokers. Paik et al. (2012) demonstrated prevalence in 12% of never-smokers versus 2% of former/current smokers. Although some studies have suggested an intrinsically poorer prognosis for patients with *ALK* rearrangement several biases may have confounded these results, and further work in this area is ongoing. However, most studies have shown that *ALK*-positive adenocarcinomas do not respond to anti-EGFR TKIs.

(b) *KRAS*

In Western countries, *KRAS* mutations have been identified in about 25% of lung adenocarcinomas. They are associated with resistance to gefitinib or erlotinib, and have a poor prognosis. They are less prevalent in East Asian populations. Ninety-five per cent of *KRAS* mutations occur in codons 12–13 and tend to be observed in smokers. A study of 481 lung adenocarcinomas identified *KRAS* mutations in 15% of never-smokers and 47% of ex-/current smokers. No clinical demographic differences were observed compared with patients with wild-type *KRAS*. In never-smokers, *KRAS* mutations tend to be observed in mucinous invasive adenocarcinomas with a lepidic pattern (formerly called bronchioloalveolar carcinomas). *KRAS* and *EGFR* mutations tend to be mutually exclusive.

8. Are there any drugs that are currently licensed for any of these indications?

Crizotinib is an ATP-competitive inhibitor of ALK, MET, RON, and ROS1 kinases. It was being developed in phase I trials as a MET inhibitor when NSCLC *ALK* rearrangements were identified and development was subsequently restricted to *ALK*-rearranged NSCLC. It achieved accelerated Food and Drug Administration (FDA) approval for treatment of *ALK*-positive locally advanced or metastatic NSCLC after phase I and II trials demonstrated impressive response rates of 54–61% in *ALK*-positive NSCLC, disease control rates of 90%, and PFS of 10 months. Phase III trials comparing crizotinib with pemetrexed or docetaxel in the second-line setting, and with cisplatin–pemetrexed in the first-line setting will quantify the magnitude of benefit from crizotinib.

> *The patient was commenced on treatment with gefitinib at the standard daily dose of 250mg with the addition of zolendronic acid every 4 weeks. Her tumour was sent for further molecular analysis as part of an on-going study. No codon 12–13 KRAS mutations, exon 15 BRAF mutations, or ALK rearrangements were detected.*

Treatment and follow-up

The patient was last reviewed 4 months into treatment with gefitinib. She attained an excellent clinical and radiological response. Her only current symptom is grade 1 anorexia. She is pain free and off opiates. Her cough has completely resolved and her ECOG performance status is 1. An up-to-date staging CT scan shows an ongoing partial remission across all disease sites.

Learning points

In NSCLC:

- testing for *EGFR* mutations is critical in therapeutic decision-making;
- smoking history is critical to determining likelihood of *EGFR* mutation present;
- patients whose tumours have known *EGFR* mutations should have first-line treatment with a TKI (gefitinib or erlotinib) over platinum-doublet chemotherapy;
- crizotinib is FDA approved for *ALK*-rearranged relapsed NSCLC; European Medicines Agency approval is awaited;
- *KRAS* mutations are well recognized in never-smokers and are associated with a poor prognosis and lack of response to gefitinib or erlotinib;
- *KRAS* and *EGFR* mutations are relatively mutually exclusive.

Further reading

Couraud S, Zalcman G, Milleron B, Morin F, Souquet P-J. Lung cancer in never smokers—a review. *European Journal of Cancer* 2012; **48**: 1299–1311.

Lee JS, Park K, Kim S-W, et al. A randomized phase III study of gefitinib (IRESSA®) versus standard chemotherapy (gemcitabine plus cisplatin) as a first-line treatment for never-smokers with advanced or metastatic adenocarcinoma of the lung. *Journal of Thoracic Oncology* 2009; 4 (9 Suppl 1): 283.

Maemondo M, Inoue A, Kobayashi K, et al. Gefitinib or chemotherapy for non–small-cell lung cancer with mutated EGFR. *New England Journal of Medicine* 2010; **362**: 2380–2388.

Mitsudomi T. Erlotinib, gefitinib, or chemotherapy for EGFR mutation-positive lung cancer? *Lancet Oncology* 2011; **12**: 710–711.

Mok TS, Wu Y-L, Thongprasert S, et al. Gefitinib or carboplatin-paclitaxel in pulmonary adenocarcinoma. *New England Journal of Medicine* 2009; **361**: 947–957.

Paik PK, Johnson ML, D'Angelo SP, et al. Driver mutations determine survival in smokers and never-smokers with stage IIIB/IV lung adenocarcinomas. *Cancer* 2012; **118**: 5840–5847.

Rosell R, Carcereny E, Gervais R, et al. Erlotinib versus standard chemotherapy as first-line treatment for European patients with advanced EGFR mutation-positive non-small-cell lung cancer (EURTAC): a multicentre, open-label, randomised phase 3 trial. *Lancet Oncology* 2012; **13**: 239–246.

Rudin CM, Avila-Tang E, Harris CC, et al. Lung cancer in never smokers: molecular profiles and therapeutic implications. *Clinical Cancer Research* 2009; **15**: 5646–5661.

Scagliotti G, Stahel RA, Rosell R, Thatcher N, Soria J-C. ALK translocation and crizotinib in non-small cell lung cancer: an evolving paradigm in oncology drug development. *European Journal of Cancer* 2012; **48**: 961–973.

Shepherd FA, Rodrigues Pereira J, Ciuleanu T, et al. Erlotinib in previously treated non-small-cell lung cancer. *New England Journal of Medicine* 2005; **353**: 123–132.

Thatcher N, Chang A, Parikh P, et al. Gefitinib plus best supportive care in previously treated patients with refractory advanced non-small-cell lung cancer: results from a randomised, placebo-controlled, multicentre study (Iressa Survival Evaluation in Lung Cancer). *The Lancet* 2005; **366**: 1527–1537.

Yang JC-H, Shih J-Y, Su W-C, et al. Afatinib for patients with lung adenocarcinoma and epidermal growth factor receptor mutations (LUX-Lung 2): a phase 2 trial. *Lancet Oncology* 2012; **13**: 539–548.

Zhou C, Wu YL, Chen G, et al. Erlotinib versus chemotherapy as first-line treatment for patients with advanced EGFR mutation-positive non-small-cell lung cancer (OPTIMAL, CTONG-0802): a multicentre, open-label, randomised, phase 3 study. *Lancet Oncology* 2011; **12**: 735–742.

Case 6

Single brain metastasis from breast cancer

Thankamma Ajithkumar

Case history

A 51-year-old woman presented to the emergency department with a 5-day history of increasing headache and drowsiness. She had had no significant illnesses in the past. All blood tests were normal. She had a CT scan followed by a MRI scan of the brain (Fig. 6.1).

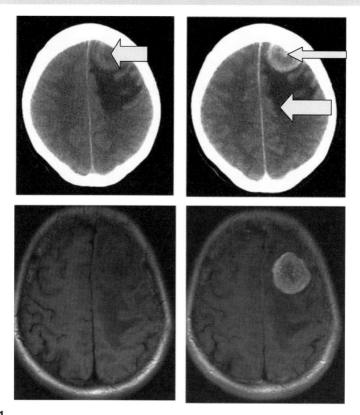

Fig. 6.1

Question

1. What do the CT and MRI scans show in Fig. 6.1?

Answer

1. What do the CT and MRI scans show in Fig. 6.1?

The CT scan shows a well-defined peripheral hyperdense tumour over the left frontal region, which enhances uniformly. It has a broad base along the frontal bone
with no evidence of thickening of the underlying bone (hyperostosis). There is surrounding oedema and mass effect with effacement of the lateral ventricle. The MRI
scan shows a hypointense well-defined lesion in the frontal region which enhances
with no areas of necrosis. There is associated oedema. The differential diagnoses
of a well-defined lesion in the brain with contrast enhancement are meningioma,
high-grade brain tumour, lymphoma, and metastasis. As meningioma is slow growing, oedema is not a common associated feature (except in the anaplastic variant),
so the oedema in this case raises the suspicion of a high-grade brain neoplasm or
metastasis.

Subsequently this patient underwent a complete macroscopic excision of the brain lesion. Histology showed a poorly differentiated adenocarcinoma, which on immuno-histochemical staining was positive for CK7 and epithelial membrane antigen (EMA), and negative for ER and PgR receptors, CK20, and TTF-1.

Questions

2. How do you interpret the immunohistochemistry?
3. How would you investigate further?

Answers

2. How do you interpret the immunohistochemistry?

Histology shows a poorly differentiated adenocarcinoma. The common primary sites are lung, breast, and the gastrointestinal system. Immunohistochemistry using CK7, CK20, and TTF-1 is useful for identifying the primary tumour. TTF-1 helps to distinguish pulmonary from non-pulmonary adenocarcinoma. TTF-1 is positive in 81% of lung cancers and 69% of metastatic lung cancers. CK20 is not expressed in lung cancer but is positive in gastrointestinal adenocarcinoma and urothelial tumours. CK7 is not expressed in gastrointestinal cancers but is positive in lung, breast, endometrial, and ovarian cancers. A combination of CK7+/CK20– is seen in 100% of lung cancers, 88% of breast cancers, and 87% of ovarian cancers. Table 6.1 shows the various possible combinations of CK7/CK20 staining.

The combination of CK7+, CK20–, and TTF-1- in this case suggests the possibility of lung or breast cancer (the two most common primaries metastasizing to brain). TTF-1 positivity is useful to confirm lung adenocarcinoma, but a negative result cannot rule out a lung primary. Similarly, ER and PgR positivity can only point towards a hormone-positive breast cancer, but ER and PgR negativity cannot rule out a breast cancer.

Table 6.1 Correlation of primary tumours with CK7 and CK20 staining

Staining pattern	Primary tumour
CK7+/CK20+	Urothelial, pancreas, biliary, stomach
CK7+/CK20–	Lung, breast, ovary, pancreas, biliary
CK7–/CK20+	Colon, stomach
CK7–/CK20–	Prostate, kidney, liver

3. How would you investigate further?

The immunohistochemistry suggests a possible lung or breast cancer with ovarian, pancreatic, or biliary cancer being less likely alternatives. Since there is a possibility of this being a HER-2-positive breast cancer, the HER-2 status needs to be assessed.

The primary tumour site can be established in half of patients presenting with brain metastases from an unknown primary. Hence further radiological staging investigations with CT scan of the chest, abdomen, and pelvis are needed to identify a possible primary tumour. Some studies suggest that there is little value in routine mammography or breast imaging in patients with brain metastases of unknown primary because such a presentation of breast cancer is uncommon.

A CT scan of the chest, abdomen, and pelvis was unremarkable except for a 13mm right axillary lymph node. A mammogram showed a small area of asymmetric increased parenchymal density in the right upper inner quadrant suspicious of a malignancy. This lesion was unchanged compared with a screening mammogram taken 6 months previously. However, an ultrasound guided biopsy from the parenchymal density showed a grade 2 invasive carcinoma staining positive for E-cadherin, HER-2/neu, and GCDFP-15. Meanwhile, the pathologist had reported the brain lesion to be HER-2/neu 3+. The patient subsequently underwent a PET scan which showed uptake in the right axillary lymph node, T11 and L5 vertebrae, and the left sacroiliac joint.

Questions

4. What is the significance of staining with E-cadherin and GCDFP-15?
5. Do you advise any further treatment to the brain?
6. What would be your approach to the management of breast cancer in this woman?
7. If your treatment includes trastuzumab, for how long would you recommend it?
8. How will you assess the response and what would be your follow-up plan?

Answers

4. What is the significance of staining with E-cadherin and GCDFP-15?

E-cadherin distinguishes lobular from ductal carcinoma. A negative E-cadherin stain confirms lobular carcinoma (specificity 97.7%; negative predictive value 96.8%; sensitivity 88.1%; positive predictive value 91.2%) whereas ductal carcinomas invariably stain positive with E-cadherin. GCDFP-15 is a useful marker for identifying metastatic breast cancer in the absence of previous history of breast cancer and/or in tumours which are negative for ER and PgR. It has a specificity of 95% and sensitivity of 74%. Positivity for both these stains hence suggests primary breast cancer (as opposed to metastasis to the breast) of ductal origin.

5. Do you advise any further treatment to the brain?

This patient had a complete macroscopic excision of the brain metastasis. The role of post-operative radiotherapy after complete excision of a tumour is debatable. One randomized trial of 95 patients compared immediate post-operative whole-brain radiotherapy with observation and salvage whole-brain radiotherapy at progression. The study showed improved surgical bed and distant recurrence rates (10 and 18% versus 46 and 70%) with immediate radiotherapy, but without an improvement in OS. However, this study was not powered to detect any improvement in OS (Patchell et al. 1998). A retrospective study of stereotactic radiosurgery to the resection cavity showed an actuarial local control rate of 79% at 1 year (Soltys et al. 2008).

In summary, there is no definite evidence for advocating routine post-operative radiotherapy after complete resection of a solitary metastasis. Nevertheless, many clinicians recommend post-operative whole-brain radiotherapy giving a dose of 25–30Gy in 10–15 fractions.

6. What would be your approach to the management of breast cancer in this woman?

This woman has a histologically proven small-volume metastatic breast cancer with a completely excised brain metastasis. Patients with one to five metastatic lesions usually limited to a single organ are often referred to as having oligometastatic disease. It has been estimated that 1–10% of newly diagnosed oligometastatic breast cancers can be 'cured' (Hanrahan 2005) with an aggressive approach involving surgery, radiotherapy, and systemic treatment. Since this patient has metastasis in more than one organ, this case is not one of oligometastatic disease but just low-volume metastatic disease. The clinical challenges in this case are, thus, to decide the optimal systemic therapy (whether trastuzumab alone or in combination with chemotherapy) and its duration, and to define the role of loco-regional therapy.

The options for first-line treatment in this patient include single-agent trastuzumab or a combination of chemotherapy with trastuzumab. The optimal systemic treatment for metastatic breast cancer is not known. The choice is between sequential single agents and combination chemotherapy. In the majority of patients the overall survival with single-agent systemic agents is equivalent to that with combination chemotherapy. The decision regarding the choice of initial treatment depends on various patient-related factors such as menopausal status, ECOG performance status, patient preference, etc., and disease-related factors such as HER-2 status, ER/PgR status, tumour burden, and the need for rapid disease and/or symptom control (Cardoso et al. 2009). For patients in whom speedy disease control is not warranted (i.e. those without life-threatening visceral metastases and/or rapidly progressive disease) sequential single-agent treatment is preferred.

In HER-2-positive patients, a number of studies have shown that the addition of trastuzumab to chemotherapy results in high rates of response and better PFS and overall survival than chemotherapy alone. However, it is not known whether the addition of chemotherapy to trastuzumab improves outcome in HER-2-positive patients compared with trastuzumab alone. The only study of this is a randomized phase II trial comparing trastuzumab plus docetaxel with sequential trastuzumab followed by docetaxel at progression (Hamberg et al. 2011). This small study of 101 patients showed a similar PFS in both arms (9.4 months in the combination arm and 9.9 months in the sequential one). The objective response rate was better with combination therapy (79 vs. 53%, $P = 0.016$). Overall survival was non-significantly shorter in the sequential arm (30.5 vs. 19.7 months, $P = 0.11$).

Since this patient has low-volume metastases without life-threatening or rapidly progressive disease, single-agent treatment with trastuzumab is an acceptable choice.

The role of loco-regional treatment in metastatic breast cancer is not known. Retrospective studies suggest that resection of the primary tumour in metastatic breast cancer improves OS and median PFS. This benefit may be attributable to a reduced tumour burden and/or to better accessibility of systemic treatment. However, it cannot be routinely recommended (Pockaj et al. 2010).

7. If your treatment includes trastuzumab, for how long would you recommend it?

The optimal duration of trastuzumab monotherapy in metastatic breast cancer is unknown. Many clinicians prefer to recommend treatment until progression, in the absence of toxicity, or if patient wishes to discontinue.

8. How will you assess the response and what would be your follow-up plan?

Methods for assessing response include clinical examination, imaging, and serial assays of cancer antigen 15-3 (CA15-3) and CEA. However, tumour markers need to be used carefully as levels can rise ('flare') during the first 2 months of treatment. Similarly, bone scans may also show a 'healing flare' in the initial months which can persist for as long as 12 months. Follow-up should be tailored to the individual clinical needs.

Treatment and follow-up

This patient received whole-brain radiotherapy (30Gy in 10 fractions) followed by 3-weekly trastuzumab as a single agent. Re-staging after 4 years showed no evidence of recurrence or progression of brain disease, and stable disease in other sites. She continues on trastuzumab with no side-effects.

Further reading

Brown PD, Asher AL, Farace E. Adjuvant whole brain radiotherapy: strong emotions decide but rational studies are needed. *International Journal of Radiation Oncology Biology Physics* 2008; **70**: 1305–1309.

Cardoso F, Bedard PL, Winer EP, et al. International guidelines for management of metastatic breast cancer: combination vs sequential single-agent chemotherapy. *Journal of the National Cancer Institute* 2009; **101**: 1174–1181.

Hamberg P, Bos MM, Braun HJ, et al. Randomized phase II study comparing efficacy and safety of combination-therapy trastuzumab and docetaxel vs. sequential therapy of trastuzumab followed by docetaxel alone at progression as first-line chemotherapy in patients with HER2+ metastatic breast cancer: HERTAX trial. *Clinical Breast Cancer* 2011; **11**: 103–113.

Hanrahan EO, Broglio KR, Buzdar AU, et al. Combined-modality treatment for isolated recurrences of breast carcinoma: update on 30 years of experience at the University of Texas M.D. Anderson Cancer Center and assessment of prognostic factors. *Cancer* 2005; **104**: 1158–1171.

Pagani O, Senkus E, Wood W, et al. International guidelines for management of metastatic breast cancer: can metastatic breast cancer be cured? *Journal of the National Cancer Institute* 2010; **102**: 456–463.

Patchell RA, Tibbs PA, Regine WF, et al. Postoperative radiotherapy in the treatment of single metastases to the brain: a randomized trial. *Journal of the American Medical Association* 1998; **280**: 1485–1489.

Pockaj BA, Wasif N, Dueck AC, et al. Metastasectomy and surgical resection of the primary tumor in patients with stage IV breast cancer: time for a second look? *Annals of Surgical Oncology* 2010; **17**: 2419–2426.

Soltys SG, Adler JR, Lipani JD, et al. Stereotactic radiosurgery of the postoperative resection cavity for brain metastases. *International Journal of Radiation Oncology Biology Physics* 2008; **70**: 187–193.

Case 7

Breast cancer at a nuclear power station

Adrian Harnett

Case history

A 36-year-old Russian security guard at Sizewell nuclear power station presented to her GP with a lump in her left breast. There was no nipple discharge or distortion. She had not had any lumps in the past. She had two children aged 5 and 3 who had been breast-fed for about 11 months. She was seen with her English husband, also a security guard at the power station. Mammography followed by core biopsy confirmed malignancy.

Question

1. What is unusual about this case?

Answer

1. What is unusual about this case?

The patient is young, under 40, and so it is important to enquire about a family history of breast cancer.

Her grandmother on her father's side had breast cancer in her 60s and she is now 85. Her grandfather's sister had breast cancer in her 50s and died at the age of 85.

She has worked at Sizewell for 8 years as a security officer on the main gate. She has no relevant past medical history, is not on any medication, and is a non-smoker.

Question

2. What does this information indicate?

Answer

2. What does this information indicate?

Although two of her relatives had breast cancer, they were not close relatives and developed cancer after the menopause so it is unlikely that she has a *BRCA1* or *-2* mutation. It is interesting to note that both lived on to old age so did not have particularly aggressive breast cancers. Her employment at Sizewell is extremely unlikely to have had any role in the aetiology, because if she had had any increased radiation exposure it would have been at a very low level and it would be most unusual for it to cause a breast cancer within the short timescale of 8 years. However, records monitoring her radiation exposure should be checked and confirmation sought that she had not been exposed to any radiation incidents.

A mastectomy and axillary clearance were performed. Histopathology revealed a 51mm grade II invasive ductal carcinoma with associated intermediate ductal carcinoma in situ (DCIS) (see Fig. 7.1A). There was intermediate-grade DCIS and a background of in situ lobular neoplasia and also pseudo-angiomatoid stromal hyperplasia (PASH) (Fig. 7.1B). This latter feature is not uncommon in breast specimens but tends to be seen in younger patients. Ibrahim et al. (1989) found microscopic foci of PASH in 23% of 200 consecutive breast specimens obtained for benign and malignant conditions, 89% of which were from patients younger than 50 years.

Lymphovascular invasion was present. Margins were clear but 3/14 lymph nodes were involved and extracapsular invasion was seen. The tumour was strongly ER receptor positive and HER-2 negative.

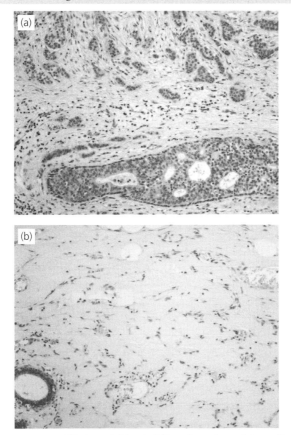

Fig. 7.1 (images courtesy of Dr Joseph Murphy) (See also colour plate section)

Questions

3. Is this result surprising?
4. What course of action would you recommend?

Answers

3. Is this result surprising?

Breast cancer in patients aged under 40 is more likely to be high grade and HER-2 positive (particularly if BRCA negative). Fewer cancers are hormone receptor positive in the under 40s than the over 40s. The nodal involvement is not surprising, but it is unusual to have such a large grade II ductal carcinoma. Lobular carcinomas tend to be more diffuse. The histopathology should be reviewed.

In summary, this was a conventional mammary carcinoma with no particular features to suspect it was radiation induced.

4. What course of action would you recommend?

In view of the young age of the patient and the large tumour, staging investigations including CT and bone scans should be performed.

Staging investigations did not reveal any evidence of distant metastatic disease.

Question

5. Is there any other line of enquiry that should be pursued?

Answer

5. Is there any other line of enquiry that should be pursued?

It should be noted that the patient is Russian. Enquiry should be made into her upbringing and when she came to the UK. More details about her family should be sought.

She lived 200 to 300km south of Chernobyl and left the area when she finished school in 1989. She was 14 when the nuclear accident occurred there. Neither she nor her family were evacuated at the time; in fact they learnt of the accident 15 months later. Her younger sister, who was also exposed to radiation from Chernobyl, died of a brain tumour at the age of 3.

Question

6. What further management would you recommend?

Answer

6. What further management would you recommend?

Firstly you would have to explain that the radiation incident at Chernobyl is highly likely to have caused her breast cancer, as well as the brain tumour in her younger sister. This could also explain the slightly unusual pathology as discussed in the answer to Question 2.

Reassurance should be given about her treatment to date and that the surgery she has completed has been a large component of that treatment. It has removed most if not all of the cancer and the scans give reassurance in that there is no evidence of distant spread. However, she is at risk of developing recurrence later due to the presence of undectable microscropic disease, and the risk of this can be significantly reduced by giving adjuvant treatment.

Adjuvant chemotherapy using a combination regime was given. She received eight courses of FEC chemotherapy (5-FU, epirubicin, and cyclophosphamide) and on completion was commenced on tamoxifen. She was given post-operative radiotherapy to the left chest wall and supraclavicular fossa (40Gy in 15 fractions over 3 weeks) to reduce the risk of loco-regional relapse because she had a large, node-positive tumour with lymphovascular invasion in the primary tumour and extracapsular invasion in the nodes.

Questions

7. In retrospect does she fulfil the criteria for neoadjuvant chemotherapy?
8. Discuss the advantages and disadvantages of neoadjuvant chemotherapy.

Answers

7. In retrospect does she fulfil the criteria for neoadjuvant chemotherapy?

The tumour was more diffuse and larger histologically than the pre-operative examination and imaging had suggested. Neoadjuvant chemotherapy would have been a very reasonable alternative management option if the extent of disease had been appreciated before surgery. Neoadjuvant chemotherapy is indicated for:

- locally advanced and inflammatory breast cancer—where it should be the standard of care;
- T2 and T3 tumours where it is acceptable and preferable to routine post-operative adjuvant chemotherapy.

It is reasonable to give neoadjuvant chemotherapy to any patient who needs adjuvant chemotherapy.

8. Discuss the advantages and disadvantages of neoadjuvant chemotherapy.

The advantages of neoadjuvant chemotherapy outweigh the disadvantages: some are obvious and some are theoretical but we shall discuss them together.

Advantages:

- It increases the breast conservation rate due to tumour regression.
- It can make inoperable tumours suitable for mastectomy.
- It can measure marker lesions to monitor the response to chemotherapy, unlike with adjuvant treatment.
- Systemic treatment makes sense, treating any nodal or microscopic disease early when the breast primary is still *in situ*.
- The tumour is less viable and tumour shedding at surgery is reduced if neoadjuvant therapy is employed.
- Recent studies have confirmed an overall survival benefit for neoadjuvant therapy.
- Forty per cent of positive axillary nodes convert to negative nodes after neoadjuvant therapy.

Disadvantages:

- Histology is only available from a core biopsy, so from a limited amount of tissue, but more importantly it does not take account of tumour heterogeneity.
- There is no surgical staging.
- You may not know where the tumour is! It is important to be prepared for success, to know where the tumour is, and how to image it.
- You can get a response that leaves residual multifocal disease spread over the same area that was involved prior to chemotherapy.

One year after completion of treatment she is well and clinical examination is unremarkable. She wishes to have a breast reconstruction.

Questions

9. How would you advise her?
10. What other factors should be discussed with the patient?

Answers

9. How would you advise her?

It is entirely reasonable and understandable that she wishes to have breast reconstruction. She has coped with all her treatment well and has no evidence of recurrent disease. If the breast cancer does relapse this is most likely to occur in a few years' time as the tumour was hormone receptor positive. It is probably unreasonable to expect her to wait some years before considering reconstruction. The surgical options are reduced as she has had post-operative radiotherapy. A tissue expander technique is contraindicated as the elasticity of the irradiated skin and tissues will have been considerably compromised.

10. What other factors should be discussed with the patient?

It is important the patient is as fit as possible, not overweight, and a non-smoker. The usual recommendation is a body mass index of less 30 (kg/m²) and ideally less than 27. Failure of the reconstruction is far more likely to happen in smokers because of compromised vasculature. Several consultations are often necessary in preparation for breast reconstruction, involving not only specialist nurses and physiotherapists but also dieticians and, when appropriate, smoking cessation clinics.

Progress and follow-up

The patient was referred for breast reconstruction, which was carried out after weight reduction and without complication (Fig. 7.2). She has been very pleased with the result and continues to remain well on follow-up 4½ years after the original diagnosis.

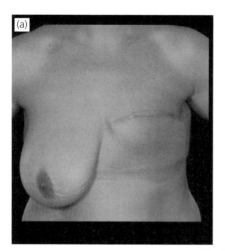
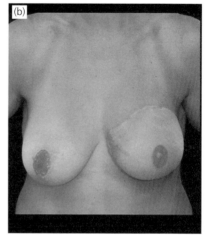

Fig. 7.2

Further reading

Hortobagyi G. William L. McGuire Memorial Lecture: neoadjuvant systemic therapy: promising experimental model, or improved standard of care? *Cancer Research* 2012; 72(24 Suppl): abstract ML-1.

Ibrahim RE, Sciotto CG, Weidner N. Pseudoangiomatous hyperplasia of mammary stroma. Some observations regarding its clinicopathologic spectrum. *Cancer* 1989; **63**: 1154–1160.

Case 8

Oesophagus

Tom Roques

Case history

A 65-year-old man presents with a 3-month history of increasing dysphagia—initially to solids but increasingly to liquids too. He has lost 15kg in weight (20% of his baseline). He has a background of severe rheumatoid arthritis for which he has been on methotrexate for 7 years. He is referred on a 2-week wait suspected cancer pathway and has an endoscopy which shows a tight malignant-looking stricture from 25 to 29cm. Biopsies show a moderately differentiated squamous cell carcinoma.

Questions

1. What initial staging tests should be performed?
2. How should his weight loss be managed while these tests are carried out?

Answers

1. What initial staging tests should be performed?

Staging investigations are performed to decide whether the tumour is localized to the oesophagus and adjacent nodes and therefore potentially curable and, if there are no metastases, to assess local extent and suitability for resection or radiation. A CT scan of the chest, abdomen, and pelvis with intravenous contrast and oral water is the first imaging test performed. Axial slices should be 2.5–5mm thick to allow multiplanar reformatting which can be particularly helpful in showing/refuting invasion into adjacent organs. If this shows potentially curable disease, a [18]FDG PET-CT scan and endoscopic ultrasound (EUS) assessment should also be attempted. EUS may not be possible if the tumour is stricturing. The information from each of these investigations and the diagnostic endoscopy is complementary, but EUS is the most sensitive for assessing local invasion (T stage). A bronchoscopy may be helpful for mid-oesophageal cancers if there is possible invasion of the carina or bronchial tree. EUS is the most sensitive investigation for nodes close to the tumour, but PET-CT has higher specificity and sensitivity for more distant nodal disease. PET-CT will reveal unsuspected metastatic disease in up to 30% of patients at presentation, but it has 5% false positive and false negative rates so solitary hot spots should be correlated with other diagnostic tests.

2. How should his weight loss be managed while these tests are carried out?

This patient has malnutrition (>10% weight loss over 3–6 months) which may compromise his ability to tolerate potentially curative treatment. A dietician should assess him urgently and discuss his calorie intake. A liquidized high-calorie diet and high-protein drinks will be recommended. If, despite these recommendations, he continues to lose weight, nasogastric feeding should be instituted. Careful monitoring of electrolytes in the first few days of nasogastric feeding will help to prevent re-feeding syndrome. A covered plastic stent that could later be removed can also be considered.

The CT scan shows circumferential thickening of the oesophagus over 5cm and an 8mm para-oesophageal lymph node at the superior extent of the tumour. At EUS three suspicious para-oesophageal nodes are seen—all adjacent to the primary tumour which is 4.5cm long and extends into the muscularis but not beyond the oesophagus. The PET-CT scan shows avid uptake of tracer in the mid-oesophagus over 6cm (SUV = 19) but without evidence of nodal spread. None of the investigations show distant metastases.

Questions

3. What stage is the tumour?
4. What are the curative treatment options?

Answers

3. What stage is the tumour?

T3N2M0 using the 7th edition of the AJCC staging manual (the 6th edition is still used in some centres—in which case this tumour would be T3N1 as there are only N0, N1, and Nx nodal staging categories in the older version).

4. What are the curative treatment options?

Several combination treatments are possible for T3N2 disease though there is a paucity of phase III data comparing different options. Clinical trial data are also hampered by broad inclusion criteria (site and histology) and, in the case of radiotherapy, by evidence based on obsolete treatment techniques.

Surgery is the basis for most curative treatments if the patient is fit enough. A two-stage Ivor Lewis oesophagectomy is the usual technique, but minimally invasive oesophagectomy is becoming more widespread. Neoadjuvant chemotherapy with two cycles of cisplatin and 5-FU improves 5-year survival from 17.1% to 23% (Allum et al. 2009). Radiotherapy alone has a small chance of cure, but combined chemotherapy and radiation has cure rates similar to those of surgically based options, although the two approaches have not been compared in adequately powered studies. Whether radiation with concomitant chemotherapy should also be preceded by chemotherapy is uncertain. Triple-modality therapy—chemoradiation followed by surgery—is another option but again there is a paucity of data to support it, though further studies are ongoing. This approach should be considered if the patient is being treated by a multidisciplinary team (MDT) experienced in such therapy. Given all the uncertainties, patients should be offered the chance to participate in clinical trials where possible. The final treatment decision should be taken by the MDT, reflecting local expertise with the involvement of the patient's perspective, priorities, and wishes. If chemotherapy is used, a dose reduction should be considered in view of his prior treatment with methotrexate which may affect his bone marrow reserve.

The patient declines surgery on the basis that a close friend died shortly after an oesophagectomy some years before. A potentially curative regime of two cycles of neo-adjuvant chemotherapy with cisplatin and 5-FU followed by definitive chemoradiation is agreed. He tolerates chemotherapy well and has a good response both symptomatically and on imaging. The radiotherapy planning CT scan shows the axial bulk of the tumour to be reduced and that the tumour is now 4cm long.

Questions

5. How should the gross tumour volume (GTV), clinical target volume (CTV), and planning target volume (PTV) be defined?
6. What dose of radiation should be prescribed?

Answers

5. How should the gross tumour volume (GTV), clinical target volume (CTV_, and planning target volume (PTV) be defined?

The tumour GTV (GTV-T) should be defined using the maximum extent of tumour on all available initial investigations (endoscopy, CT, EUS, and PET-CT). In this case the GTV-T should extend over 6cm (the PET-CT length). The nodal GTV (GTV-N) should be defined separately to include all adjacent oesophageal nodes (as highlighted on EUS). Many historical radiotherapy protocols generate a CTV by expanding the GTV with 5cm longitudinal margins for most of the treatment course with a reduced volume for a second phase. There is now good evidence to support the use of a single-phase technique with reduced longitudinal margins as this technique does not seem to produce marginal recurrences.

To define the CTV-T, the GTV-T should initially be extended 20mm superiorly and inferiorly along the plane of the oesophagus. This volume is then isometrically expanded by a 10mm margin in the axial plane. GTV-N is expanded by 10mm in all dimensions to produce a CTV-N. The two CTVs are summed and then edited to reflect likely patterns of tumour spread (e.g. into adjacent para-oesophageal nodes even if not radiologically involved) and natural barriers to local invasion (e.g. edited off the spinal column, aorta, and lungs). The CTV–PTV expansion margin should be defined according to local audit but will be in the region of 5mm axially and 10mm in the longitudinal plane.

6. What dose of radiation should be prescribed?

Several radiation doses have been used in clinical trials: 50Gy in 25 fractions combined with chemotherapy is a UK standard and was used in the recently completed SCOPE trial. Higher doses (up to 65Gy) have been used in some studies but there is no evidence that dose escalation is advantageous.

The patient completes treatment successfully and is eating a soft diet without the need for supplements 2 months later. Eighteen months after radiotherapy he has further difficulty in swallowing.

Questions

7. What are the two most likely diagnoses?
8. How should they be treated?

Answers

7. What are the two most likely diagnoses?

The two most likely diagnoses are a radiation-induced stricture, which occurs in approximately 20% of patients after definitive chemoradiation, or recurrent cancer.

8. How should they be treated?

A radiation-induced stricture is best managed by regular endoscopic dilatations together with nutritional advice from a dietician. Recurrent cancer should be confirmed histologically. The patient should be staged again to see whether this recurrence is local or metastatic. If there is no distant disease salvage surgery could be considered, but the benefit of this is uncertain with the likelihood of cure very low and the complication rate relatively high. Local palliation with brachytherapy or a stent should be considered. Palliative chemotherapy should be discussed with the patient but supportive and palliative care are the most important things to consider.

Treatment and follow-up

At endoscopy a tight stricture at 28cm was seen and successfully dilated. Biopsies of the strictured region did not show cancer. He remains well 35 months after chemoradiation but has needed further dilatation on two occasions.

Further reading

Allum WH, Stenning SP, Bancewicz J, et al. Long-term results of a randomized trial of surgery with or without preoperative chemotherapy in esophageal cancer. *Journal of Clinical Oncology* 2009; 27: 5062–5067.

Allum WH, Blazeby JM, Griffin SM, et al. Guidelines for the management of oesophageal and gastric cancer. *Gut* 2011; 60: 1449–1472.

Button MR, Morgan CA, Crotdon ES, et al. Study to determine adequate margins in radiotherapy planning for esophageal carcinoma by detailing patterns of recurrence after definitive chemoradiotherapy. *International Journal of Radiation Oncology Biology Physics* 2009; 73: 818–823.

Van Hagen P, Hulshof MC, van Lanschot JJ, et al. (the CROSS Group). Preoperative chemoradiotherapy for esophageal or junctional cancer. *New England Journal of Medicine* 2012; 366: 2074–2084.

Case 9

Stomach

Tom Roques

Case history

A 56-year-old man is admitted with an episode of haematemesis and a haemoglobin level of 97g/L. An endoscopy shows a 5cm malignant-looking ulcer in the pre-pyloric region of the stomach. Biopsies from the ulcer confirm a poorly differentiated mucinous type adenocarcinoma. He has type 2 diabetes and hypertension, which are both well controlled on oral medication. He is discharged home with a plan to complete his staging investigations as an outpatient.

Question

1. What staging investigations should be requested and why?

Answer

1. What staging investigations should be requested and why?

A contrast-enhanced CT scan of the chest, abdomen, and pelvis with intravenous contrast and oral water should be performed to assess local extent, lymphadenopathy, and to look for distant metastases. If this scan confirms disease localized to the stomach and adjacent nodes the patient should have a staging laparoscopy. This will assess both the primary tumour (and in particular whether there is invasion of local organs), the number and size of local lymph nodes, and the presence or absence of peritoneal disease and liver metastases. Any suspicious peritoneal or liver nodules should be biopsied. EUS is unlikely to add more information to laparoscopic staging. PET-CT is not routinely recommended as many gastric cancers (particularly those of the mucinous type) do not take up FDG so false negative rates are relatively high.

These tests confirm a T3N2 cancer without clear evidence of peritoneal, liver, or more distant spread. The patient meets a surgeon who feels he has operable disease and is healthy enough to undergo surgery.

Question

2.   Assuming he is well enough for all oncological treatments, what two curative approaches could be considered and what is the evidence for each?

Answer

2. Assuming he is well enough for all oncological treatments, what two curative approaches could be considered and what is the evidence for each?

The standard approach in the UK would be to use perioperative chemotherapy—three cycles of epirubicin, cisplatin, and capecitabine (ECX) (or epirubicin, cisplatin, and infusional 5-FU; ECF) before surgery and another three afterwards. The MAGIC study randomized 503 patients, 74% of whom had stomach cancer, to surgery alone or surgery with perioperative ECF chemotherapy. Five-year survival improved from 23 to 36% with the addition of chemotherapy. The REAL-2 study showed that substituting capecitabine for infusional 5-FU produced equivalent results in advanced oesophago-gastric cancers. Extrapolating this to the perioperative setting, ECX has therefore become a standard perioperative chemotherapy regime.

An alternative would be to operate initially and to follow this with adjuvant chemoradiotherapy, an approach favoured in the United States. The evidence for this comes from the Intergroup 0116 trial which randomized 556 patients to surgery alone versus surgery and adjuvant radiochemotherapy (45Gy in 25 fractions plus 5-FU and leucovorin) and showed an improvement in 5-year survival from 23 to 42%. This approach is not usually favoured in the UK, particularly because of concerns about the large numbers of patients having less than D1 resection in the trial and the toxicity of the radiotherapy.

He completes three cycles of preoperative ECF chemotherapy with grade 3 diarrhoea after the second cycle necessitating a 3-day admission to hospital for rehydration. His capecitabine dose is reduced to 75% thereafter. His restaging CT after three cycles shows a reduction in volume of the primary tumour but also a small pulmonary embolus.

Question

3. How should the pulmonary embolus be managed?

Answer

3. How should the pulmonary embolus be managed?

The management of incidental pulmonary emboli on chemotherapy is relatively controversial and without a strong evidence base, but this patient is about to undergo surgery which in itself is a risk factor for further thromboembolic events. He should therefore be anticoagulated with a therapeutic dose of low-molecular-weight heparin or rivaroxaban before surgery and warned about the possibility of further bleeding from his tumour. Assuming that the prothrombotic effect of chemotherapy is partly the cause, treatment dose low-molecular-weight heparin should be continued for the duration of adjuvant treatment and for a total of up to 6 months. There is insufficient evidence to recommend the placement of an inferior vena cava filter prior to surgery in an asymptomatic pulmonary embolus but it should be considered in the event of a symptomatic event.

He has a resection of his tumour and recovers well from his surgery. Pathology shows a good response to chemotherapy (Mandard grade 3; see Box 9.1) and he commences post-operative chemotherapy but is admitted with neutropenic sepsis after his second cycle and does not complete a third. He remains well for 17 months until he presents with abdominal pain and weight loss of 5kg in a month. A re-staging CT confirms the presence of peritoneal metastases and moderate-volume ascites as well as multiple liver metastases measuring up to 23mm in diameter. His original tumour is tested for HER2 by immunohistochemistry and found to be 3+. His ECOG performance status is 1.

Box 9.1 Pathological assessment of tumour regression after preoperative chemotherapy

Mandard tumour regression grades (TRG)

TRG 1: Complete regression—absence of residual cancer and fibrosis extending through the different layers of the oesophageal/stomach wall.

TRG 2: Presence of rare residual cancer cells scattered through the fibrosis.

TRG 3: An increase in the number of residual cancer cells, but fibrosis still predominates.

TRG 4: Residual cancer outgrowing fibrosis.

TRG 5: Absence of regressive changes.

Reproduced from Madard AM, et al. Pathologic assessment of tumor regression after preoperative chemoradiotherapy of esophageal carcinoma: clinicopathologic correlations. *Cancer* 1994; **73**(11): 2680–2686. Copyright © 1994 American Cancer Society, with permission from John Wiley and Sons, Inc. All Rights Reserved.

Question

4. Which chemotherapy regimen would you recommend and why?

Answer

4. Which chemotherapy regimen would you recommend and why?

Trastuzumab, cisplatin, and capecitabine (TCX), based on evidence from the ToGA trial (Bang et al. 2010) (though this study recruited chemo-naïve patients), National Institute for Health and Care Excellence (NICE) guidance, and the relatively long disease-free interval from ECX and previous response to this regime. Up to six cycles should be given depending on response. This should be followed by maintenance trastuzumab until disease progression.

Question

5. What regular monitoring, in addition to standard pre-chemotherapy blood tests, should be performed?

Answer

5. What regular monitoring, in addition to standard pre-chemotherapy blood tests, should be performed?

Echocardiogram to assess left ventricular ejection fraction in view of treatment with trastuzumab and CT scan of the chest, abdomen, and pelvis to assess response, each every 3 months.

He has stable disease on imaging after three cycles of chemotherapy but is admitted after the fifth cycle with increasing abdominal distension. A CT confirms large-volume ascites and progression of his liver metastases. Five litres of ascitic fluid is drained and his chemotherapy is stopped. On review 3 weeks later the ascites has reaccumulated.

Question

6. What are the options for management of his ascites?

Answer

6. What are the options for management of his ascites?

The ascites is likely to continue to reaccumulate quickly and need management for the rest of his life. A peritoneal drain could be inserted as and when it becomes symptomatic, but this would mean repeated hospital visits. A permanent tunnelled peritoneal catheter could be inserted under ultrasound control. This could then be drained by the patient or his carer at home using a vacuum bottle, reducing the need for recurrent hospital attendances. The patient should be offered entry into early phase clinical trials if he is well enough, but there is no standard chemotherapy option with an evidence base in this situation.

Treatment and follow-up

A tunnelled catheter was inserted and palliated his ascites to good effect. He continued to deteriorate at home and died there 10 weeks later.

Further reading

Bang YJ, Van Cutsem E, Feyereislova A, et al. Trastuzumab in combination with chemo-therapy versus chemotherapy alone for treatment of HER2-positive advanced gastric or gastro-oesophageal junction cancer (ToGA): a phase 3, open-label, randomised controlled trial. *The* Lancet 2010; **376**: 687–697.

Cunningham D, Allum WH, Stenning SP, et al. Perioperative chemotherapy versus surgery alone for resectable gastroesophageal cancer. *New England Journal of Medicine* 2006; **355**: 11–20.

Cunningham D, Starling N, Rao S, et al. Capecitabine and oxaliplatin for advanced esophago-gastric cancer. *New England Journal of Medicine* 2008; **358**: 36–46.

Hurt CN, Nixon LS, Griffiths GO, et al. SCOPE1: a randomised phase II/III multicentre clinical trial of definitive chemoradiation, with or without cetuximab, in carcinoma of the oesopha-gus. *BMC Cancer* 2011; **11**: 466.

Macdonald JS, Smalley SR, Benedetti J, et al. Chemoradiotherapy after surgery compared with surgery alone for adenocarcinoma of the stomach or gastroesophageal junction. *New England Journal of Medicine* 2001; **345**: 725–730.

NICE. *Gastric cancer (HER2-positive metastatic) – trastuzumab.* NICE Technology Appraisal Guidance 208, November 2010.

NICE. *The PleurX peritoneal catheter drainage system for vacuum assisted drainage of treatment-resistant recurrent malignant ascites.* NICE Medical Technology Guidance 9, March 2012.

Case 10

Neuroendocrine tumour

Gaurav Kapur

Case history

A 67-year-old man with a long-standing history (dating back 9 years) of recurring hypoglycaemic attacks, was referred by his GP. His earlier symptoms had been relieved when he was given glucose. More recently, the symptoms had progressed both in frequency and severity—the patient developed symptoms of diarrhoea, abdominal pain, and nocturnal cramps. In view of this, his GP had commenced him on mebeverine and temazepam. A Boehringer Mannheim (BM) test gave an average blood glucose monitoring result of 2mmol/L. The full blood count (FBC), liver function tests, and urea and electrolytes (U&Es) were normal. Table 10.1 shows the results of a 48-h fast.

Table 10.1 Results of the 48-h fast

Insulin	84pmol/L	(0–60)
C-peptide	1757pmol/L	(174–960)
Fasting glucose	2.0mmol/L	(3.5–7.0)
Sulfonylurea screen	Negative	

Questions

1. What is your provisional diagnosis?
2. How would you investigate the case further?

Answers

1. What is your provisional diagnosis?

Insulinoma. The diagnostic criteria for insulinoma, called the Whipple triad, are

- symptoms of hypoglycaemia
- plasma glucose ≤2.2mmol/L
- relief of symptoms with glucose.

The diagnosis is confirmed by inappropriately high levels of insulin during a spontaneous or induced episode of hypoglycaemia.

A 72-h fast does not normally produce symptomatic hypoglycaemia due to a hormonally mediated increase in glucose production. However, if there is any defect in the ability to maintain normoglycaemia, such as an excess of insulin, a prolonged fast will result in hypoglycaemia. Though 72-h fast has been the standard test for the diagnosis of insulinoma, one study suggests that a 48-h fast is sufficient to make a diagnosis.

The fast is ended when the plasma glucose concentration is ≤45mg/dl (2.5mmol/L), the patient has symptoms or signs of hypoglycaemia, 72 h have elapsed, or when the plasma glucose concentration is less than 55mg/dl (3mmol/L) if the Whipple triad was documented on a previous occasion.

At the end of the fast 1mg of glucagon is given intravenously and plasma glucose is measured at 10, 20, and 30 min post-administration.

The European Neuroendocrine Tumor Society (ENETS) guidelines recommend the presence of the following criteria in addition to symptoms to make a diagnosis of insulinoma:

1. documented blood glucose levels ≤2mmol/L
2. concomitant raised insulin levels of ≥36pmol/L
3. C-peptide levels of ≥200pmol/L
4. pre-insulin levels ≥5pmol/L
5. beta-hydroxybutarate levels ≤2.7 mmol/L
6. absence of sulfonylurea in the plasma or urine.

A plasma insulin concentration of 20.8pmol/L when the plasma glucose concentration is below 3.0mmol/L is consistent with hyper-insulinaemia (e.g. insulinoma).

Plasma C-peptide distinguishes endogenous from exogenous hyperinsulinaemia. Normal subjects who are hypoglycaemic will have lower values. Because of the antiketogenic effect of insulin, plasma beta-hydroxybutyrate concentrations are lower in patients with insulinoma than in normal subjects.

Sulfonylureas are only present in the plasma in hypoglycaemia induced by oral hypoglycaemic agents.

Insulin is antiglycogenolytic and hyperinsulinaemia allows for the retention of glycogen within the liver. Therefore, patients with insulin-mediated hypoglycaemia respond to the administration of 1mg of intravenous glucagon (a glycogenolytic agent) by releasing glucose. Normal subjects will have released virtually all glucose from the liver at the end of the 72-h fast and cannot respond as vigorously to intravenous glucagon as a patient with an insulinoma. At the end of the fast, patients with an insulinoma have an increase in plasma glucose of 1.4mmol/L or more in 20 to 30 min, whereas normal subjects have a smaller increment.

2. How would you investigate the case further?

Once a diagnosis of an insulinoma is suspected, staging scans with a CT abdomen ± EUS of the pancreas should be performed.

Questions

3. What does the CT scan show (Fig. 10.1)?
4. How do you proceed?

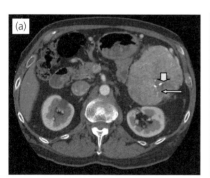 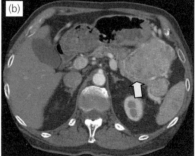

Fig. 10.1

Answers

3. What does the CT scan show (Fig. 10.1)?

There is a large (8cm × 8cm) avidly enhancing mass lying within the left peritoneal cavity, with some central necrosis (thin arrow-figure 10.1a) and calcification (thick arrow-figure 10.1a) Multiple lateral large vessels are seen passing through the mass (arrow-figure 10.1b). The mass is abutting many retroperitoneal and intraperitoneal structures but is not obviously arising from them.

4. How do you proceed?

A biopsy of the mass should be performed to confirm the diagnosis.

*A core biopsy of the mass was performed. This showed sheets and interconnecting tra-
beculae of polygonal cells in which there are round to oval nuclei and abundant eosin-
iphilic granular cytoplasm with an extensive fine vascular stromal network. The cells
stained positively for CD56 and chromogranin but were negative for TTF-1.*

Question

5. How would you interpret the histology and immunohistochemistry. What is
   the unifying diagnosis?

Answer

5. How would you interpret the histology and immunohistochemistry. What is the unifying diagnosis?

This is a neuroendocrine tumour, not arising from the lung. The unifying diagnosis would be an insulinoma.

The immunohistochemocal markers of neuroendocrine tumours are CD56, synaptophysin, and chromogranin. Histological features of the tumour do not usually correlate with the anatomical sites or hormone production, but if amyloid deposition is noted on histopathological assessment it often indicates an insulin-secreting pancreatic neuroendocrine tumour. TTF-1 is a marker for lung tumours, and in the absence of any other supporting evidence is useful for excluding a bronchial origin for the tumour.

The patient underwent a distal pancreatectomy and splenectomy. The post-operative histology confirmed the diagnosis of neuroendocrine tumour. The study of tumour proliferation indices showed a Ki-67 index of 2–5% and four mitoses per high-power field (HPF).

Questions

6. What does the Ki-67 index indicate?
7. Would you advise any post-operative treatment?

Answers

6. What does the Ki-67 index indicate?

The Ki-67 protein is a cellular marker for proliferation, and is present during all active phases of the cell cycle (G_1, S, G_2, and mitosis) but is absent from resting cells (G_0). These values indicate that this is a well-differentiated tumour. The Ki-67 index also correlates with survival (high values indicate a poorer prognosis).

Mitotic activity is a measure of the proliferative potential, and along with the Ki-67 index is used for grading purposes. The optimal cut-off values for both Ki-67 and mitoses/HPF have not been established. Table 10.2 shows the current ENETS classification.

Table 10.2 The ENETS classification

Differentiation	Ki-67	Mitosis/10HPF
Well differentiated	≤2%	<2
Moderately differentiated	3–20	2–20
Poorly differentiated	>20	>20

Adapted with permission from Rindi G, et al. TNM staging of foregut (neuro)endocrine tumors: a consensus proposal including a grading system. *Virchows Archiv: the European Journal of Pathology* **449**: 395–401. Copyright © Springer-Verlag 2006.

7. Would you advise any post-operative treatment?

The patient was put on a surveillance programme with 3-monthly clinic reviews, with a history, clinical exam, and tumour markers [chromogranin A, urinary 5-hydroxyindoleacetic acid (5-HIAA)] at each visit, CT imaging at 6-monthly visits, and an annual octreotide scan. Haemoglobin A1C levels were checked at each visit to obtain an understanding of his glycaemic control, with other tests such as insulin to be done if clinically indicated.

Nine months later he developed recurrent symptoms of hypoglycaemic attacks and abdominal discomfort. Insulin levels were 46mmol/L, with elevated chromogranin A levels. He had re-staging with a CT scan and an octreotide scan (Fig. 10.2).

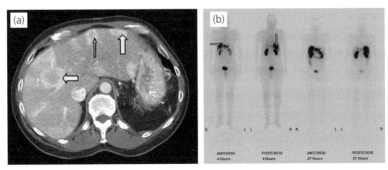

Fig. 10.2

Questions

8. What do these scans show?
9. What further management would you institute at this point?

Answers

8. What do these scans show?

There are multiple enhancing intrahepatic lesions characteristic of metastases from a neuroendocrine carcinoma. These tumours are highly vascular (A) and may appear isodense with the liver during certain contrast phases. They generally enhance intensely with intravenous contrast during the early arterial phases of imaging, with washout during the delayed portal venous phase. The octreotide scan shows avidity in most sites of metastatic disease (B).

9. What further management would you institute at this point?

Given the avid disease on octreotide scan, the appropriate treatment would be a somatostatin analogue (octreotide LAR 20mg 4-weekly).

Somatostatin analogues (growth hormone-inhibitory hormone) inhibit the release of various peptide hormones in the gut, pancreas, and pituitary, antagonize growth factor effects on tumour cells, and, at very high doses, may induce apoptosis. Whilst octreotide is highly effective in controlling the symptoms associated with glucagonomas, VIPomas, and carcinoid tumours, it is less predictable for symptomatic patients with insulinoma. Nevertheless, it is a reasonable choice for patients with persistent hypoglycaemia that is refractory to diazoxide. In this case the patient refused treatment with diazoxide due to concerns over certain side-effects of the drug, and therefore was commenced on octreotide LAR.

Diazoxide is an antihypertensive agent with hyperglycaemic effects, and is usually effective in controlling symptoms of hypoglycaemia in patients with insulinomas. Adverse effects include oedema, hirsuitism, weight gain, and renal dysfunction. There are two commercially available long-acting somatostatin analogues:

Sandostatin LAR—given in doses of 10, 20, or 30mg, every 4 weeks as a deep intramuscular injection

Lanreotide—given in doses of 60, 90, or 120mg every 4 weeks as a deep subcutaneous injection.

The patient responded well to somatostatin analogues for 2 years, with no further hypoglycaemic episodes, normalization of bowel movements, and good reduction in chromogranin A levels. Average blood glucose levels were around 4.5mmol/L. However, after 2 years there was clinical, biochemical, and radiological evidence of progression.

Question

10. What are the further treatment options?

Answer

10. What are the further treatment options?

The treatment options include:

◆ radionuclide targeted therapy

◆ streptozotocin- or temozolomide-based chemotherapy

◆ new agents such as sunitinib (tyrosine kinase inhibitor) or everolimus [a mammalian target of rapamycin (mTOR) inhibitor].

Targeted radionuclide therapy is useful for patients with inoperable or asymptomatic neuroendocrine tumours and has become a standard of care in the UK and Europe. The radiolabels of choice are yttrium-90 and lutetium-177. The most commonly used peptides include DOTA-TOC and DOTA-TATE.

At 6–8-week intervals, 3–6GBq of ^{90}Y-DOTA-TOC or ^{90}Y-DOTA-TATE is administered to a cumulative dose of 12–18GBq. Most patients report subjective benefits, often with improved tumour markers, within two treatment cycles. At 6–10-week intervals, 3.7–7.4GBq of ^{177}Lu-DOTA-TATE is administered to cumulative activities of 22–29.6GBq. Partial response rates of 28% and minor response rates/stable disease in 54% have been reported. In more recent trials streptozotocin-based chemotherapy regimens resulted in a response rate of 36–38%.

Sunitinib and everolimus are licensed for the use in advanced and progressive well-differentiated pancreatic neuroendocrine tumours. Sunitinib, at a dose of 37.5mg orally per day, has been shown to double PFS from 5.5 to 11.4 months. Everolimus has improved PFS from 4.6 to 11.0 months compared with placebo.

The patient opted for treatment with targeted radionuclide therapy. He was assessed and found suitable for treatment with ^{177}*Lu-DOTA-TATE. He received four treatments at 2-monthly intervals. Post-treatment he was found to have stable disease radiologically, with a good biological and clinical response (haemoglobin A1C 5.8%).*

Eighteen months later he had evidence of further disease progression, with a significant increase in the size of the retroperitoneal lesions, and new deposits in the liver. He was not considered to be suitable for further radionuclide therapy due to a suboptimal GFR and was commenced on therapy with sunitinib.

Question

11. What other aspect of treatment should you consider in this patient?

Answer

11. What other aspect of treatment should you consider in this patient?

A referral to a clinical geneticist should be made. Neuroendocrine tumours may occur as part of familial endocrine cancer syndromes such as multiple endocrine neoplasia type 1 (MEN1), MEN2, neurofibromatosis 1, von Hippel–Lindau disease, and Carney complex (see Fig. 10.3). Although most are sporadic, 5% of insulinomas are associated with MEN1 and should therefore be referred for genetic screening.

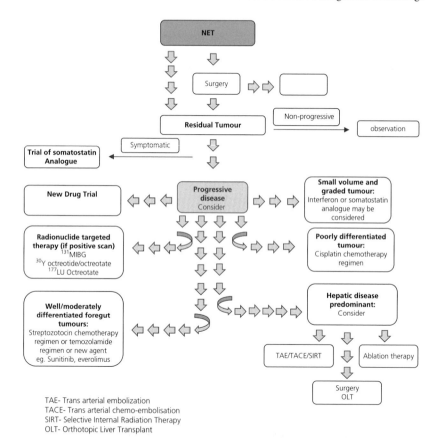

TAE- Trans arterial embolization
TACE- Trans arterial chemo-embolisation
SIRT- Selective Internal Radiation Therapy
OLT- Orthotopic Liver Transplant

Fig. 10.3 UKI NETS (UK and Ireland Neuroendocrine Tumour Society) algorithm for treatment of neuroendocrine tumours.

Reproduced from Ramage et al, An international peer-reviewed journal for health professionals and researchers in gastroenterology and hepatology, GUT, Volume 61, Issue 1, pp. 6–32, Copyright © 2012, with permission from BMJ Publishing Group Ltd.

Further reading

Ramage JK, et al. Guidelines for the management of gastroenteropancreatic neuroendocrine (including carcinoid) tumours (NETs). *Gut* 2012; **61**: 6–32.

Case 11

A patient presenting with painless jaundice

Elizabeth Liniker, Simon Johnston, Sara Custodio-Cabello, and Bristi Basu

Case history

A 51-year-old woman presented with a short history of painless jaundice. She had no significant past medical history and was not on any regular medications. She was otherwise well with an ECOG performance status of 0. On clinical examination her abdomen was soft and non-tender with no palpable masses. Blood test results were as follows: FBC, U&Es, calcium, clotting profile all normal; bilirubin 112μmol/L; alkaline phosphatase 387U/L; alanine aminotransferase (ALT) 267U/L; gamma-glutamyltransferase 245U/L; albumin 34g/L; CA 19.9—169U/ml (normal value 0–39). The patient had a contrast enhanced CT of the chest, abdomen, and pelvis (Fig. 11.1). She underwent an EUS-guided fine-needle aspiration biopsy of the pancreas. Subsequent cytology revealed cytological atypia (nuclear enlargement) in keeping with at least high-grade dysplasia.

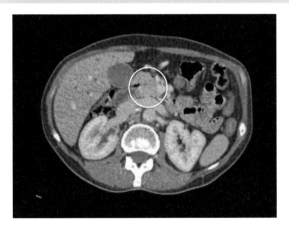

Fig. 11.1

Questions

1. What does Fig. 11.1 show?
2. Outline your management if there were no distant metastases evident on staging imaging.

Answers

1. What does Fig. 11.1 show?

Axial contrast enhanced images of the abdomen show a mass in the head of the pancreas with biliary dilatation.

In light of a mass in the head of the pancreas and highly suggestive histology, the diagnosis is adenocarcinoma of the pancreas causing biliary obstruction. Histological confirmation is occasionally difficult in these tumours because of the surrounding stromal reaction. However, they often show positive immunohisto-chemical staining for CK19, CA19.9, and CEA.

2. Outline your management if there were no distant metastases evident on staging imaging.

The first question is does she have resectable disease which could be potentially cured with surgery. Fewer than 20% of patients have resectable tumours at diagnosis, 30–40% have locally advanced unresectable disease, and the remainder have metastases at presentation. Given that if the patient has a good performance status and no significant comorbidities to contraindicate major surgery, determination of resectability is appropriate and should be assessed using:

♦ Diagnostic imaging: triple-phase contrast-enhanced thin-slice (multidetector row) CT is the gold standard staging investigation and predicts resectability in 80–90% of patients.

♦ EUS: the presence or absence of vascular invasion can be visualized using EUS. In cases where small pancreatic tumours are suspected, EUS is able to detect these with a greater sensitivity than CT, MRI, or FDG-PET.

♦ Laparoscopy: in selected cases, where there is a higher than usual index of suspicion for occult metastases (e.g. a very high CA19.9 at diagnosis), laparoscopy may be performed to try to detect occult liver and peritoneal metastases.

Although distant spread represents an unambiguous contraindication to resection, there are differing opinions as to when a pancreatic cancer is technically resectable and when an attempt at resection is appropriate. In general, major arterial involvement (superior mesenteric, coeliac, and common hepatic arteries) remains a contraindication to resection due to the high risk of involved (R1) margins post-operatively and therefore an increased risk of loco-regional recurrence. However, the presence of short segment portal vein or superior mesenteric vein involvement no longer constitutes an absolute contraindication to resection due to the increasing use of vascular resection and grafts. In recognition of this fact, recently a new category of 'borderline resectability' has emerged (Table 11.1).

In the pre-operative setting, biliary drainage is only indicated in patients with cholangitis, those with significant liver dysfunction, and those who are symptomatic, such as with severe pruritus. Studies show that routine pre-operative biliary drainage for individuals with obstructive jaundice has a worse outcome than resection alone.

Table 11.1 Resectablility criteria for pancreatic cancer

Affected vessel	Resectable	Borderline resectable
SMA	Clear surrounding fat plane	Tumour abutment affecting ≤180° of circumference of vessel wall
Coeliac axis or hepatic artery	Clear surrounding fat plane	Gastroduodenal artery encasement up to hepatic artery with either: • short segment encasement or • direct abutment of hepatic artery without extension into coeliac axis
SMV–PV	No evidence of: • tumour abutment • distortion • tumour thrombus • venous encasement	Presence of: • tumour abutment • encasement of SMV–PV without arterial encasement • short segment venous occlusion but with suitable vessel proximal and distal allowing for safe resection and reconstruction

SMA, superior mesenteric artery; SMV-PV, superior mesenteric vein–portal vein.

Question

3. What is the evidence for adjuvant chemotherapy after resection?

Answer

3. What is the evidence for adjuvant chemotherapy after resection?

Even completely resected (R0) pancreatic cancers have a poor prognosis, with 5-year survival rates in the range of 10–25% and median survival between 10 and 20 months. So a great proportion of patients who are currently regarded as resectable will have occult metastatic disease at the time of surgery. For those patients who undergo resection and remain fit, the current standard of care is to offer 6 months of adjuvant systemic chemotherapy. The ESPAC-1 and CONKO-001 (Oettle et al. 2007) trials demonstrated a significant benefit in 5-year survival (from <10% to around 20%) with adjuvant 5-FU/folinic acid and adjuvant gemcitabine, respectively, with the ESPAC-3 study then showing equivalence in survival between adjuvant gemcitabine and 5-FU/folinic acid (Neoptolemos et al. 2010). Current trials are evaluating whether there is additional benefit from the addition of agents such as capecitabine to gemcitabine. A new approach yet to be proven in large clinical trials may be to consider neoadjuvant treatment strategies. The period of neoadjuvant treatment may identify patients with early progression who are unlikely to benefit from upfront surgery with its associated morbidity and may also evaluate the feasibility of downstaging borderline unresectable disease to enable an R0 resection.

The patient underwent a laparotomy with a view to Whipple's resection. However, at surgery, her disease was found to be inoperable on the basis of invasion of the common hepatic artery, which had been understaged by her diagnostic imaging. A palliative gastro-jejunostomy and hepatico-jejunostomy bypass was therefore performed. She made a very good postoperative recovery and her bilirubin normalized.

Question

4. What approaches to further treatment could you take in this case?

Answer

4. What approaches to further treatment could you take in this case?

In the absence of resectable disease, palliative treatments should be discussed with the patient. The optimal management plan for patients with locally advanced, unresectable pancreatic cancer is controversial and median survival in these cases is in the range of 6–10 months. Commonly used approaches involve chemotherapy, as for metastatic disease, or chemoradiation.

Gemcitabine is considered the benchmark palliative therapy following its comparison with bolus 5-FU because of an improvement in 1-year survival rate in one study (18% versus 2%) (Burris et al. 1997). There is also evidence that gemcitabine can provide symptomatic benefit with stabilization of weight and improvements in pain and performance scores. However, gemcitabine monotherapy does not provide a significant improvement in median survival duration, and unfortunately the addition of other chemotherapy drugs or targeted agents has largely not shown any additional benefit in a randomized phase III setting. A modest improvement in OS with addition of capecitabine to gemcitabine has been shown in a meta-analysis (Cunningham et al. 2009). Adding erlotinib to gemcitabine demonstrated a statistically significant improvement in OS in a randomized setting; the increase was only about 2 weeks (Moore et al. 2007).

Chemoradiotherapy can be used in locally advanced pancreatic cancer (LAPC). Phase III studies (FFCD/SFRO, ECOG) have shown that chemoradiotherapy is associated with greater toxicity than chemotherapy alone but can offer small improvements in outcomes. Different regimens and end-points (resectability, OS, local progression) have been studied without providing a definitive answer as to the optimum approach (Chauffert et al. 2008, Loehrer et al. 2011). However, given the increased toxicity of chemoradiotherapy and the early development of metastatic disease in many patients with locally advanced pancreatic cancer, there is evidence that preceding chemoradiotherapy with chemotherapy may spare those patients with rapidly progressive disease, thus selecting those patients who are most likely to benefit (Huguet et al. 2007).

The patient underwent 3 months of chemotherapy with gemcitabine plus capecitabine. Re-staging scans that showed stable disease so she was offered chemoradiation. A dose of 50.4Gy in 28 fractions with concomitant capecitabine was prescribed. A CT scan after treatment showed stable disease. However, 6 months following completion of chemoradiotherapy, she complained of right-sided abdominal pain and CT imaging revealed new liver metastases. The patient had an ECOG performance status of 1 and her blood tests were unremarkable apart from an aspartate aminotransferase (AST) of 70U/L and bilirubin of 19μmol/L.

Questions

5. What systemic therapy could be considered in this case?
6. Outline the principles of symptom control in patients such as this.

Answers

5. What systemic therapy could be considered in this case?

There is no standard chemotherapy regimen in this situation. Nevertheless, the pivotal PRODIGE 4/ACCORD 11 trial in metastatic pancreatic cancer patients, comparing first-line gemcitabine monotherapy with the FOLFIRINOX regimen demonstrated a significant advance in median OS from 6.8 months in the gemcitabine arm to 11.1 months with FOLFIRINOX (HR 0.56; 95% CI 0.45–0.73; $P < 0.001$) (Conroy et al. 2011). However, FOLFIRINOX was considerably more toxic, with more than 10% of patients experiencing grade 3/4 diarrhoea and 5.4% febrile neutropenia. The impressive response rates (31.6% versus 9.4%) seen in the trial have led to interest in evaluating this regimen in an earlier setting in the management of pancreatic cancer. However, the toxicity of the regimen necessitates careful patient selection for those with excellent performance status and fitness, limiting its role within the general population of patients diagnosed with metastatic pancreatic cancer. Therefore, wherever possible these patients should be offered enrolment into a clinical trial if they are eligible.

6. Outline the principles of symptom control in patients such as this.

Metastatic pancreatic cancer gives rise to symptoms that are challenging to palliate, and hence early referral to specialist palliative care is advised. Achieving and maintaining a good quality of life is the main aim of care, and early referral to a specialist palliative care team is recommended. Common problems such as pain, weight loss, jaundice, duodenal obstruction, ascites, and depression should be identified proactively and appropriate treatment and supportive measures instigated. Abdominal pain is a presenting symptom in 75–80% of patients. Although chemotherapy may improve pain scores, early approaches to address this should be based on the World Health Organization analgesic ladder with escalation to opiates as appropriate. Neuropathic pain from encroachment of the coeliac plexus may be targeted with medication (e.g. gabapentin) and coeliac plexus neurolysis. Cancer cachexia (weight loss >10%, anorexia, and systemic inflammation) is a typical feature of advanced pancreatic cancer. Secondary diabetes and steatorrhoea from pancreatic insufficiency may contribute to weight loss so early specialist dietetic support is recommended. Such support may help stabilize weight with institution of supplemental pancreatic enzyme replacement therapy, calories, and protein. Prokinetics such as metoclopramide may help gastric outflow obstruction (but can increase pain if there is subacute small bowel obstruction) whilst a duodenal stent may palliate duodenal obstruction. Procedures such as biliary stenting and paracentesis should be considered whenever appropriate, after careful consideration of the risk/benefit balance for such invasive measures.

Treatment and follow-up

The patient declined referral to a phase I/II clinical trial centre. Palliative care support in the community was instituted to manage her pain and fatigue. She deteriorated rapidly and died a month later.

Further reading

Burris HA 3rd, Moore MJ, Andersen J, et al. Improvements in survival and clinical benefit with gemcitabine as first-line therapy for patients with advanced pancreas cancer: a randomized trial. *Journal of Clinical Oncology* 1997; **15**: 2403–2413.

Callery MP, Chang KJ, Fishman EK, et al. Pretreatment assessment of resectable and borderline resectable pancreatic cancer: expert consensus statement. *Annals of Surgical Oncology* 2009; **16**: 1727–1733.

Chauffert B, Mornex F, Bonnetain F, et al. Phase III trial comparing intensive induction chemoradiotherapy (60 Gy, infusional 5-FU and intermittent cisplatin) followed by maintenance gemcitabine with gemcitabine alone for locally advanced unresectable pancreatic cancer. Definitive results of the 2000-01 FFCD/SFRO study. *Annals of Oncology* 2008; **19**: 1592–1599.

Conroy T, Desseigne F, Ychou M, et al. FOLFIRINOX versus gemcitabine for metastatic pancreatic cancer. *New England Journal of Medicine* 2011; **364**: 1817–1825.

Cunningham D, Chau I, Stocken DD, et al. Phase III randomized comparison of gemcitabine versus gemcitabine plus capecitabine in patients with advanced pancreatic cancer. *Journal of Clinical Oncology* 2009; **27**: 5513–5518.

Huguet F, André T, Hammel P, et al. Impact of chemoradiotherapy after disease control with chemotherapy in locally advanced pancreatic adenocarcinoma in GERCOR phase II and III studies. *Journal of Clinical Oncology* 2007; **25**: 326–331.

Loehrer PJ Sr, Feng Y, Cardenes H, et al. Gemcitabine alone versus gemcitabine plus radiotherapy in patients with locally advanced pancreatic cancer: an Eastern Cooperative Oncology Group trial. *Journal of Clinical Oncology* 2011; **29**: 4105–4112.

Moore MJ, Goldstein D, Hamm J, et al. Erlotinib plus gemcitabine compared with gemcitabine alone in patients with advanced pancreatic cancer: a phase III trial of the National Cancer Institute of Canada Clinical Trials Group. *Journal of Clinical Oncology* 2007; **25**: 1960–1966.

Neoptolemos JP, Stocken DD, Bassi C, et al. Adjuvant chemotherapy with fluorouracil plus folinic acid vs gemcitabine following pancreatic cancer resection: a randomized controlled trial. *Journal of the American Medical Association*, 2010: **304**: 1073–1081.

Oettle H, Post S, Neuhaus P, et al. Adjuvant chemotherapy with gemcitabine vs observation in patients undergoing curative-intent resection of pancreatic cancer: a randomized controlled trial. *Journal of the American Medical Association* 2007; **297**: 267–277.

Vincent A, Herman J, Schulick R, Hruban RH, Goggins M. Pancreatic cancer. *The Lancet* 2011; **13**: 607–620.

Case 12

Colon cancer

Debashis Biswas and Thankamma Ajithkumar

Case history

A 57-year-old woman presented with 2 days of abdominal pain and vomiting. On examination she had a distended abdomen with absent bowel sounds. There was no significant past medical history. Abdominal X-ray was suggestive of small bowel obstruction. Her CT scan is shown in Fig. 12.1 (no intravenous contrast was given due to previous history of allergy).

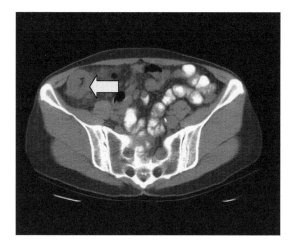

Fig. 12.1

Questions

1. What does the CT scan show?
2. Outline your initial approach.

Answers

1. What does the CT scan show?

The CT scan shows a caecal mass and appearances consistent with transmural spread and possibly serosal involvement. There are six enlarged mesocolic lymph nodes (not shown). There is no evidence of liver, peritoneal, or any other metastases.

2. Outline your initial approach.

Up to 16% of patients with colorectal cancer present with bowel obstruction. Emergency surgery in these patients is associated with significant morbidity (e.g. stoma formation) and mortality, particularly in the elderly. For example, mortality in patients aged ≥65 years having emergency surgery is 17% compared with 7.7% for those having an elective operation. The optimal management of obstructed colon cancer depends not only up on the patient's age but also on the general condition of patient, tumour location, and integrity of the bowel wall. Initial treatment options include:

◆ Segmental resection with primary anastomosis with or without proximal diversion. This is the preferred option provided there is no diffuse peritonitis or perforation and the patient is medically stable. This approach is more suitable for right-sided cancers, as in the case illustrated.

◆ (Sub)total colectomy with primary anastomosis. This is an option in left-sided obstructing tumours where there is associated with loss of bowel wall integrity or the colon proximal to the obstruction cannot be evaluated and synchronous lesions cannot be ruled out (these occur in up to 15% of patients).

◆ Resection of tumour without an anastomosis and with an end colostomy (Hartmann resection). This is an approach in left-sided tumours and allows for elective evaluation of the proximal colon with a potential for bowel preservation.

◆ Proximal colostomy only. This is carried out in medically unstable patients, as it allows for improvement in their general condition and consideration of subsequent neoadjuvant treatment.

◆ Stenting. This is an interim measure in distal colonic obstruction to restore luminal patency while awaiting full staging and allowing time for surgical optimization. Stents are less frequently used in proximal colonic obstruction as most lesions can be managed with one-stage operation and anastomosis without the need for a formal bowel preparation. However, a recent Cochrane Review suggested that in acute malignant colonic obstruction stenting has no advantage compared with emergency surgery in terms of either morbidity or mortality.

Since this patient has a right-sided tumour with small bowel obstruction, she can be managed with an emergency one-stage operation without significant anticipated risk of post-operative morbidity.

She underwent a right hemicolectomy. The pathology confirmed a grade 3 K-ras wild-type adenocarcinoma of the caecum with extramural vascular invasion and clear excision margins. Seven out of 12 lymph nodes showed metastases, including the apical group.

Questions

3. What is the stage of her disease?
4. Would you advise adjuvant treatment?
5. How do you follow her up?

Answers

3. What is the stage of her disease?

pT3N2Mx R0 according to the AJCC TNM system (7th edition) and stage C2 according to the Dukes staging system (as the apical node was involved).

4. Would you advise adjuvant treatment?

In node-positive (stage III) colon cancer 5-FU-based adjuvant chemotherapy for 6 months improves 5-year OS by 10–15% (Marsoni 2001). Studies show that oral capecitabine is an effective alternative to 5-FU plus leucovorin (Twelves et al. 2005) .

The addition of oxaliplatin to 5-FU improves survival further, especially in stage III patients aged less than 65 years. The MOSAIC study showed that the addition of oxaliplatin improved 5-year disease-free survival (DFS) by 7% (André et al. 2009). In addition, the 6-year OS in stage III patients was improved by 4%. The NSABP C-07 study confirmed this clinical benefit. The XELOXA study, which compared capecitabine plus oxaliplatin with 5-FU plus leucovocin in stage III colon cancer, showed that capecitabine plus oxaliplatin improves 3-year DFS by 4.4% (Haller et al. 2011). However, a subset analysis of the MOSAIC study suggests that patients older than 65 years do not benefit from the addition of oxaliplatin. Similarly, the ACCENT group database analysis suggests that patients aged over 70 years do not benefit from 5-FU-based chemotherapy (McCleary et al. 2013). Thus, the choice between 5-FU or capacitabine, and whether to combine this with oxaliplatin, depends on the patient's age and fitness, their predicted tolerance of each regime, and individual patient choice.

The combination of cetuximab with chemotherapy improves survival in patients with metastatic colorectal cancer whose tumours express wild-type *K-ras*. However, in stage III resected colon cancer, adjuvant treatment with cetuximab plus chemotherapy does not improve DFS (NCCTG N0147 trial), and therefore is not recommended.

The two useful web-based tools to calculate relative risk of disease-recurrence and mortality are Adjuvant! Online (<http://www.adjuvantonline.com>) and Mayo Clinic Adjuvant Tools (<http://www.mayoclinic.com/calcs/>). Using Adjuvant! Online the estimated 5-year survival of this patient is 40%, which will be improved by 22.6% with adjuvant oxaliplatin plus 5-FU/leucovorin. Therefore she was recommended to have adjuvant combination chemotherapy with capecitabine and oxaliplatin for 6 months.

5. How do you follow her up?

Disease relapse in colon cancer most commonly occurs within 3 years of surgery and there is evidence that early identification and treatment of recurrence improves survival. Regular follow-up is advised with clinical review and estimation of CEA every 3–6 months for 3 years and then 6–12-monthly until 5 years. A CT scan of the chest, abdomen, and pelvis should be performed annually for the first 3 years and colonoscopy is recommended 1 year after surgery and then every 3–5 years.

She received a combination of capecitabine and oxaliplatin for 6 months. Post-treatment staging CT and MRI scans are shown in Fig. 12.2.

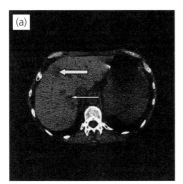 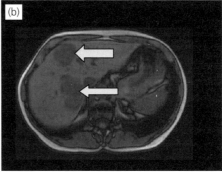

Fig. 12.2

Questions

6. What do the scans show?
7. Discuss your management.

Answers

6. What do the scans show?

The CT scan shows two hypodense areas in the right lobe of the liver suggestive of metastases (A). The MRI scan shows at least two liver lesions involving segments 7 and 8 that are hypodense on T_1-weighted images consistent with metastases (B). On T_2-weighted images the lesions are iso- to mildly heterogeneously hyperintense. The lesion in the segment 7 mildly compresses the right hepatic vein, but otherwise the hepatic veins and portal veins appear unremarkable.

7. Discuss your management.

The liver is the dominant site of metastasis in colorectal cancer, but more than two-thirds of patients with liver metastases will also have extrahepatic disease. Therefore palliative systemic chemotherapy is the treatment of choice in this situation.

In patients who present with liver as the only site of metastasis, surgical resection, when technically feasible, results in a 5-year OS of 30–35% (compared with 10% when treated with palliative chemotherapy). However, the optimal selection of patients for hepatic resection is controversial and is still evolving. Liver metastases are generally categorized as being immediately resectable, absolutely unresectable, and potentially resectable after downstaging.

Patients with immediately resectable disease have metastatic tumour with adequately resectable margins (i.e. no involvement of any major hepatic vasculature or bile ducts), no portal lymphadenopathy, absent or treatable extrahepatic disease, and adequate liver function which is likely to be preserved after resection. However, the definition of 'immediately resectable' is subjective and based to a degree on the expertise of the liver surgeon.

Patients are considered to have absolutely unresectable disease if they have non-resectable extrahepatic disease, liver failure, are unfit for surgery, or have involvement of more than 70% of the liver or six segments involved.

Approximately 12–33% of patients with isolated liver metastasis are potentially resectable after downstaging. For these patients initial systemic treatment is recommended to improve resectability.

Her case was discussed in the colorectal MDT. Although there was no extrahepatic disease on imaging, one liver metastasis was deemed to be adherent to a bile duct, and therefore her liver metastases were classified as potentially resectable after downstaging.

Question

8. Which chemotherapy regimen would you recommend?

Answer

8. Which chemotherapy regimen would you recommend?

The optimal regimen for downstaging is not known. Since there is a strong correlation between the response rate and the resection rate, a regimen with a high objective response rate is often chosen. The EORTC 40983 study showed that oxaliplatin-based chemotherapy given before and after surgery improves 3-year PFS by 9.2% compared with surgery alone for patients with liver metastasis (Nordlinger et al. 2008). However, there is no significant difference in OS between both treatments.

The addition of cetuximab to chemotherapy improves the response rate and PFS in patients with *K-ras* wild-type metastatic disease in the liver alone. The CRYSTAL trial has shown that the addition of cetuximab to irinotecan modestly improved the resection rate from 3.7 to 7% (Van Cutsem et al. 2009). In the OPUS trial, in patients with wild-type *K-ras* the addition of cetuximab increased the resectability of liver metastasis from 4 to 10% (Bokemeyer et al. 2008).

Treatment and follow-up

This woman has progressive disease immediately after oxaliplatin and capecitabine and is therefore switched to a different regimen, irinotecan plus capecitabine. Since her tumour is *K-ras* wild type, cetuximab is added to improve the chances of resection.

Further reading

André T, Boni C, Navarro M, et al. Improved overall survival with oxaliplatin, fluorouracil, and leucovorin as adjuvant treatment in stage II or III colon cancer in the MOSAIC trial. *Journal of Clinical Oncology* 2009; 27: 3109–3116.

Alberts SR, Sargent DJ, Nair S, et al. Effect of oxaliplatin, fluorouracil, and leucovorin with or without cetuximab on survival among patients with resected stage III colon cancer: a randomized trial. *Journal of the American Medical Association* 2012; 307: 1383–1393.

Bokemeyer C, Bondarenko I, Hartmann JT, et al. KRAS status and efficacy of first-line treatment of patients with metastatic colorectal cancer (mCRC) with FOLFOX with or without cetuximab: the OPUS experience. *Journal of Clinical Oncology* 2008; 26: a4000.

Cunningham D, Atkin W, Lenz H-J, et al. Colorectal cancer. *The Lancet* 2010; 375: 1030–1047.

Haller DG, Tabernero J, Maroun J, et al. Capecitabine plus oxaliplatin compared with fluorouracil and folinic acid as adjuvant therapy for stage III colon cancer. *Journal of Clinical Oncology* 2011; 29: 1465–1471.

Mahmoud N, Bullard Dunn K. Metastasectomy for stage IV colorectal cancer. *Diseases of the Colon and Rectum* 2010; 53: 1080–1092.

Marsoni S. Efficacy of adjuvant fluorouracil and leucovorin in stage B2 and C colon cancer. InternationalMulticenter Pooled Analysis of Colon Cancer Trials Investigators. *Seminars in Oncology* 2001; 28(1 Suppl 1): 14–19

McCleary NJ, Meyerhardt JA, Green E, et al. Impact of age on the efficacy of newer adjuvant therapies in patients with stage II/III colon cancer: findings from the ACCENT database. *Journal of Clinical Oncology* 2013; 31: 2600–2606.

Nordlinger B, Sorbye H, Glimelius B, et al. Perioperative chemotherapy with FOLFOX4 and surgery versus surgery alone for resectable liver metastases from colorectal cancer (EORTC Intergroup trial 40983): a randomised controlled trial. *The Lancet* 2008; **371**: 1007–1016.

Patel SS, Floyd A, Doorly MG, et al. Current controversies in the management of colon cancer. *Current Problems in Surgery* 2012; **49**: 398–460.

Twelves C, Wong A, Nowacki MP, et al. Capecitabine as adjuvant treatment for stage III colon cancer. *New England Journal of Medicine* 2005; **352**: 2696–2704.

Van Cutsem E, Köhne CH, Hitre E, et al. Cetuximab and chemotherapy as initial treatment for metastatic colorectal cancer. *New England Journal of Medicine* 2009; **360**: 1408–1417.

Case 13

Rectal cancer

Debashis Biswas and Thankamma Ajithkumar

Case history

A 47-year-old man presented with a 2-month history of increased frequency of loose bowel motions with intermittent passage of fresh rectal blood mixed with the stools. His weight had been steady, and he had a normal appetite. Digital rectal examination (DRE) revealed a low rectal mass which was tethered. The remainder of the clinical examination was unremarkable. A barium enema is shown in Fig. 13.1.

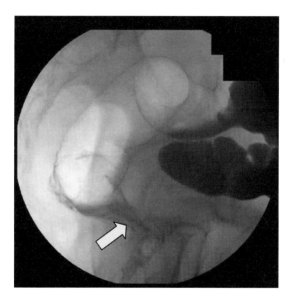

Fig. 13.1

Questions

1. What does the barium study show?
2. How would you investigate him further?

Answers

1. What does the barium study show?

The barium enema shows a large lesion in the lower rectum with mucosal ulceration suggesting a carcinoma.

2. How would you investigate him further?

Further investigations include FBC and biochemistry, colonoscopy to biopsy the mass and to exclude any synchronous tumours or polyps in the remainder of the colon, and a staging CT scan of the chest, abdomen, and pelvis. A MRI scan of the pelvis is useful for assessing the local spread of the cancer.

In patients with similar symptoms but without a palpable tumour on DRE the most appropriate initial investigation would be a procto-sigmoidoscopy.

Colonoscopy showed an ulcerative growth arising from the left lateral wall of the rectum and a pedunculated growth in the distal sigmoid colon. A biopsy confirmed a moderately differentiated adenocarcinoma of the rectum and a tubular adenoma of the sigmoid colon. There were no distant metastases. CT and MRI scans are shown in Fig. 13.2.

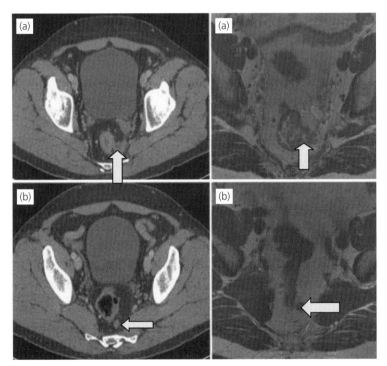

Fig. 13.2

Questions

3. What do the scans show?
4. What is the stage of his disease?
5. Outline your treatment approach.

Answers

3. What do the scans show?

The CT and MRI scans (A in Fig. 13.2) show a lesion in the rectum with extramural extension at the 4 o'clock position. The tumour is extending to involve the left lateral circumferential resection margin (CRM). Both scans (B in Fig. 13.2) show an enlarged mesorectal node at the 5 o'clock position. Other MRI images (not shown) show extension of the tumour up to the fascia of the left lateral pelvic side wall compartment posteriorly but without infiltration of the left lateral pelvic side wall.

4. What is the stage of his disease?

Radiologically the tumour extends into the left lateral CRM (T3) with an enlarged mesorectal node (N1) making the stage rT3N1M0 (rStage IIIB/Dukes C).

5. Outline your treatment approach.

Loco-regional recurrence is the predominant type of treatment failure in rectal cancer. Approximately 25% patients develop loco-regional recurrence after radical treatment. Microscopic involvement of the CRM (CRM+) is an independent predictor of local failure.

MRI scan, including a T_2-weighted image, is an essential investigation in the local staging of rectal cancer. It is useful in defining the extent of the tumour and for identifying any invasion of the mesorectal fascia (MRF) by the tumour (as in this case). MRI can also detect vascular invasion, which is a predictor of systemic recurrence. The close proximity of tumour to the MRF (as defined by a distance of $\leq 1mm$) increases the risk of a positive CRM.

Recent strategies have focused on reducing the risk of local recurrence in rectal cancer. One of the strategies is the use of pre-operative radiotherapy in patients with rectal cancer where MRI can assess the risk of CRM involvement. This helps to downstage tumours so as to enable a compete resection (R0). This patient's imaging and clinical features suggest mesorectal fascial invasion and therefore pre-operative radiotherapy should be considered to improve the chance of an R0 resection.

Questions

6. Could the need for a pre-operative treatment have been foreseen at the time of his first consultation?

7. Describe the two regimens of pre-operative treatment for rectal cancer.

8. Which regimen would you choose for this patient and why?

Answers

6. Could the need for a pre-operative treatment have been foreseen at the time of his first consultation?

Yes. DRE is important in the staging process in rectal cancer. It helps to identity a number of tumour characteristics such as size, percentage of the circumference involved, radial position, tumour level, and the level of deep fixation. Occasionally large mesorectal nodes can also be palpated. In this patient, DRE revealed that the tumour was tethered, which suggest a deeper level of invasion, and therefore the possibility of the tumour extending to the CRM.

7. Describe the two regimens of pre-operative treatment for rectal cancer.

The two evidence-based regimens of pre-operative treatment for rectal cancer are short-course radiotherapy and long-course chemoradiotherapy.

Short-course radiotherapy involves five daily doses of 5Gy followed by resection within a week of completion, whereas long-course radiotherapy delivers 45–54Gy in 25–28 fractions (usually combined with chemotherapy) followed by surgery 6–8 weeks later. Short-course radiotherapy is proven to reduce the risk of local recurrence in operable rectal cancer. The MRC-CR07 trial compared pre-operative radiotherapy with selective post-operative chemoradiotherapy in operable rectal cancer (Sebag-Montefiore 2009). At a median follow-up of 4 years, pre-operative radiotherapy resulted in a significantly lower local recurrence (4.4% versus 11%), and a better 3-year DFS (78% versus 72%) compared with selective post-operative chemoradiotherapy.

The EORTC 22921 study compared concurrent chemoradiotherapy (using 5-FU and leucovorin for 5 days during the first and fifth weeks of radiotherapy) with pre-operative radiotherapy (45Gy in 25 fractions) alone (Bosset et al. 2005). Pre-operative chemoradiotherapy resulted in a higher pathological complete response rate (14% versus 5%), and better downstaging (tumour less than pT3, 42% versus 57%). A meta-analysis has shown that pre-operative chemoradiotherapy results in a higher complete pathological response rate (12% versus 3.5%) and local control rate (16.5% versus 9.4%) than pre-operative radiotherapy alone.

In patients with T3/T4 or node-positive rectal cancer, studies show that neoadjuvant chemoradiotherapy is associated with more favourable long-term toxicity and fewer local recurrences than post-operative treatment. The German Rectal Cancer Study (Sauer et al. 2012) compared a regimen of chemoradiotherapy (50.4Gy in 28 fractions alone with 5-FU for 5 days during the first week and fifth weeks of radiotherapy) given either pre- or post-operatively. Follow-up at 10 years showed a lower risk of pelvic recurrence (7% versus 10%) with pre-operative treatment but with no survival advantage compared with post-operative treatment. Patients who received pre-operative treatment were twice as likely to undergo sphincter-sparing surgery (39% versus 19%).

The NSABP trial R-04 reported a similar efficacy of 5-FU and capecitabine with regard to complete pathological response (22% versus 19%), surgical downstaging, and sphincter preservation, along with radiotherapy (Roh et al. 2011). Therefore 5-FU and capecitabine are accepted drugs of choice in the pre-operative chemoradiotherapy regimen.

8. Which regimen would you choose for this patient and why?

This patient has a T3N1M0 rectal cancer and the MRI scan showed tumour extension into the CRM. Therefore he was recommended to have long-course radiotherapy with concomitant capecitabine chemotherapy to maximize the chance of an R0 resection.

The patient received 45Gy in 25 fractions over 5 weeks with concomitant capecitabine chemotherapy followed by a restaging CT scan and MRI scan of the pelvis. There was regression of the rectal tumour and no metastatic disease. Therefore he underwent a low anterior resection with the formation of a loop ileostomy. Histopathology showed a moderately differentiated adenocarcinoma with mucous differentiation. The tumour extended beyond the muscularis propria into the subcutaneous fat. Margins were clear. There was no evidence of vascular invasion. None of the 16 lymph nodes retrieved showed metastasis.

Questions

9. What is the post-operative staging?
10. Would you recommend further treatment, and if so what?

Answers

9. What is the post-operative staging?

ypT3N0 (0/16 lymph nodes) V0 (vascular invasion negative) R0Mx—the prefix 'y' indicates that patient had pre-operative treatment.

10. Would you recommend further treatment, and if so what?

The issue of adjuvant chemotherapy after pre-operative chemoradiotherapy in rectal cancer is controversial, and there is an on-going debate as to which patient groups may benefit from adjuvant treatment. Two trials have addressed the role of post-operative chemotherapy following pre-operative chemoradiotherapy in rectal cancer. An unplanned subset analysis of the EORTC 22921 trial showed that post-operative chemotherapy improved survival in patients whose tumours were downstaged to ypT0–2 (10% absolute DFS benefit) but not in patients whose tumours were downstaged to ypT3–4(Collette et al. 2007). A second trial from Italy showed no benefit with post-operative 5-FU-based chemotherapy.

Two current trials (the GERCOR study and ECOG–E5204) are assessing the role of post-operative chemotherapy using irinotecan and oxaliplatin-based regimens after pre-operative chemoradiotherapy in rectal cancer.

In the above patient, there was minor downstaging seen on the surgical pathology and therefore the benefit from adjuvant chemotherapy was felt to be very small.

Treatment and follow-up

This patient did not undergo adjuvant chemotherapy and remains well under surgical follow-up at 1 year.

Further reading

Bosset JF, Calais G, Mineur L, et al. Enhanced tumorocidal effect of chemotherapy with preoperative radiotherapy for rectal cancer: preliminary results—EORTC 22921. *Journal of Clinical Oncology* 2005; **23**: 5620–5627.

Collette L, Bosset JF, den Dulk M, et al. Patients with curative resection of cT3-4 rectal cancer after preoperative radiotherapy or radiochemotherapy: does anybody benefit from adjuvant fluorouracil-based chemotherapy? A trial of the European Organisation for Research and Treatment of Cancer Radiation Oncology Group. *Journal of Clinical Oncology* 2007; **25**: 4379–4386.

Glynne-Jones R, Hughes R. Critical appraisal of the 'wait and see' approach in rectal cancer for clinical complete responders after chemoradiation. *British Journal of Surgery* 2012; **99**: 897–909.

Haustermans K, Debucquoy A, Malbrecht M. The ESTRO Breuer Lecture 2010: towards a tailored patient approach in rectal cancer. *Radiotherapy and Oncology* 2011; 100: 15–21.

Kosinski L, Habr-Gama A, Ludwig K, Perez R. Shifting concepts in rectal cancer management: a review of contemporary primary rectal cancer treatment strategies. *CA: a Cancer Journal for Clinicians* 2012; **62**: 173–202.

Roh MS, Yothers GA, O'Connell MJ, et al. The impact of capecitabine and oxaliplatin in the preoperative multimodality treatment in patients with carcinoma of the rectum: NSABP R-04. [Abstract] *Journal of Clinical Oncology* 2011; **29** (Suppl 15): A-3503.

Sauer R, Liersch T, Merkel S, et al. Preoperative versus postoperative chemoradiotherapy for locally advanced rectal cancer: results of the German CAO/ARO/AIO-94 randomized phase III trial after a median follow-up of 11 years. *Journal of Clinical Oncology* 2012; **30**: 1926–1933.

Sebag-Montefiore D, Stephens RJ, Steele R, et al. Preoperative radiotherapy versus selective postoperative chemoradiotherapy in patients with rectal cancer (MRC CR07 and NCIC-CTG C016): a multicentre, randomised trial. *The Lancet* 2009; **373**: 811–820.

Anal cancer

Debashis Biswas and Thankamma Ajithkumar

Case history

A 49-year-old woman presented with a 12-month history of a painful lesion at her anus. Recently, she had been finding it difficult to evacuate her bowels because of local pain. Her general health was otherwise good. Clinical examination showed a 10cm × 8cm ulcer centred over the anus. There were no palpable inguinal lymph nodes. She declined an internal examination due to pain.

Question

1. How would you investigate further?

Answer

1. How would you investigate further?

Once a diagnosis of anal cancer is suspected, a biopsy and EUA are performed to document the extent of the tumour. In women vaginal examination should be included to screen for associated cervical cancer. A MRI of the pelvis is performed to determine the extent of local disease and a CT scan of the chest and abdomen to rule out distant metastasis.

The patient had a MRI scan (Fig. 14.1) and biopsy. Biopsy of the anal mass showed a well to moderately differentiated keratinizing invasive squamous cell carcinoma.

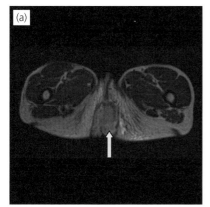 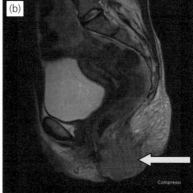

Fig. 14.1

Questions

2. What does the pelvic MRI scan show?
3. Describe the anatomy of anal canal and its lymphatic drainage.

Answers

2. What does the pelvic MRI scan show?

The MRI shows a large tumour involving the anal canal and margin (Fig. 14.1a) and displacing the posterior wall of the vagina forwards (Fig. 14.1b).

3. Describe the anatomy of anal canal and its lymphatic drainage.

The anal canal extends from the perianal region (the anal verge) to the anorectal junction. It is 3–4cm long and is divided by the dentate line. The mucosa is lined by squamous epithelium below the dentate line and by columnar epithelium above it. Tumours arising between the anorectal ring and the anal verge are classified as anal canal tumours (85%) and those arising distal to this are called anal margin tumours (15%). Lymphatics from below the dentate line drain to the inguinal and femoral nodes and subsequently to the external iliac and common iliac nodes. Above the dentate line the drainage is to the perirectal and superior rectal nodes and subsequently to the inferior mesenteric and para-aortic nodes.

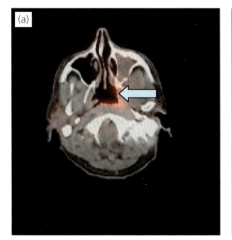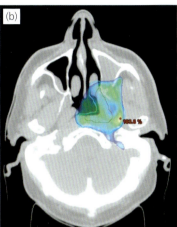

Fig. 2.2

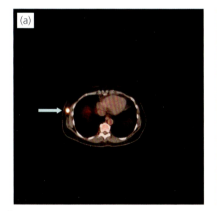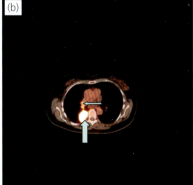

Fig. 4.2

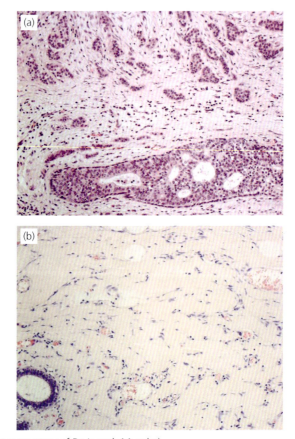

Fig. 7.1 (images courtesy of Dr Joseph Murphy)

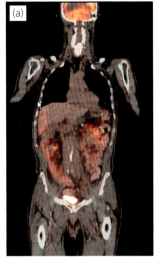
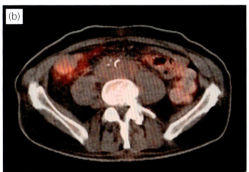

Fig. 17.3

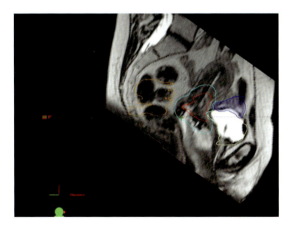

Fig. 18.2

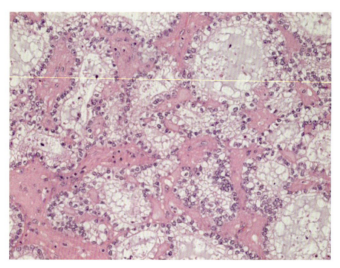

Fig. 19.2

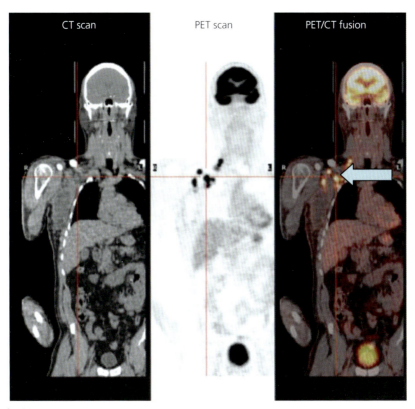

Fig. 21.1

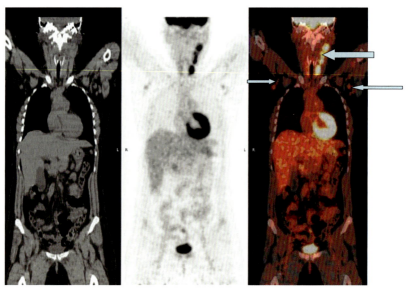

Fig. 26.1 Pre-treatment PET-CT shows activity in left cervical and bilateral axillary nodes

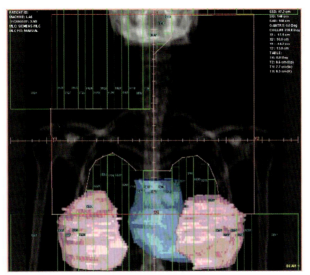

Fig. 26.2 Diagram of suggested radiotherapy field using multileaf collimator (MLC) shaping. Normal structures including the heart (centre, blue) and breasts (left and right, pink) are displayed.

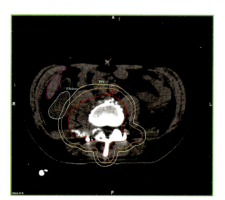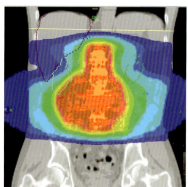

Fig. 27.2

Staging showed that the tumour extends 6 cm into the anus and measures 10cm × 8cm over the perineum. Inguinal lymph nodes were visible, but none measured more than 10mm. There were no distant metastases.

Questions

4. What is the stage of the disease?
5. What is your next step?

Answers

4. What is the stage of the disease?

rT4NxM0. Radiologically it involves the vaginal wall (T4), though inguinal nodes are visible on scan they are not assessed (Nx) and there is no metastatic disease (M0).

5. What is your next step?

She needs further investigations with PET/CT scan and histopathological examination of the inguinal nodes.

Approximately 50% of palpable or radiologically visible inguinal nodes do not contain metastasis. The incidence of inguinal nodal metastasis increases with the size of primary tumour: 0% with a tumour <2cm, 24% with a 2–5cm tumour, and 67% with a tumour >5cm. CT and MRI are less sensitive than PET/CT (62% versus 89%, respectively) in detecting inguinal node metastases, half of which are < 5mm. A PET-CT scan can have a significant impact on radiotherapy planning, especially in identifying patients who need a higher dose of radiotherapy to the groin and to rule out occult metastatic disease. PET/CT imaging changes the radiation volumes in up to 13% of patients. Therefore, it is important to rule out inguinal nodal metastasis by fine-needle aspiration cytology and/or inguinal node biopsy.

The PET scan was unsuccessful for technical reasons. Bilateral inguinal lymph node biopsies showed no evidence of malignancy.

Questions

6. What further investigations will you request?

7. Outline your treatment.

8. What common side-effects of radiotherapy would you include in the consent form?

9. What are the prognostic factors in anal cancer and what is her estimated survival?

10. How will you assess response to treatment and how will you follow her up?

11. If she were HIV positive how would you modify her treatment?

Answers

6. What further investigations will you request?

The risk factors for anal cancer include persistent infection with high-risk genotype human papilloma virus (HPV 16 is detected in 70% of anal cancers), cervical dysplasia or cancer, HIV seropositivity, smoking, anoreceptive intercourse, and immunosuppression following a solid organ transplant. There is a strong association between anal cancer and *in situ*/invasive cervical cancer so a clinical assessment of cervix, vagina, and vulva and screening for cervical and vaginal cancer should be carried out. If there is a history of possible HIV infection HIV testing is also recommended.

7. Outline your treatment.

Radical radiotherapy with concomitant chemotherapy using 5-FU and mitomycin C is the standard treatment for localized anal cancer. Primary surgery with abdominoperineal resection (APR) results in a 5-year survival of 50–70% with a local failure rate approaching 50%. Randomized phase III trials have shown that chemoradiotherapy results in a 5-year survival of 72–89% with a local failure rate of 14–37% and 5-year colostomy-free survival rate of 70–86%.

Radiotherapy is delivered in two phases as per the ACTII trial protocol giving a total dose of 50.4Gy in 28 fractions (phase I, 30.6Gy in 17 fractions; phase II, 19.8Gy in 11 fractions).

The GTV consists of the primary tumour and involved lymph nodes, which are contoured on the planning CT scan. The phase I PTV is defined by the following borders:

- superior border 1–2cm above the inferior aspect of the sacroiliac joint or 3cm above the upper limit of the known macroscopic disease (if there are pelvic nodes on the scans or the primary tumour extends to within 3cm of this border);
- lateral border, lateral to the acetabulum and covering both inguinal node regions;
- inferior border 3cm below the anal margin (for disease confined to the anal canal) or 3cm below the most inferior extent of tumour (for anal margin tumours).

The PTV for phase II consists of the GTV with 3cm margin in all directions.

8. What common side-effects of radiotherapy would you include in the consent form?

Radiation dermatitis is inevitable and can necessitate gaps in the treatment or premature discontinuation of therapy in severe cases. Diarrhoea and urinary symptoms (dysuria and frequency) are also common. Late toxicities include anal ulceration, stenosis, and necrosis necessitating a colostomy in up to 10% of patients. Patients can develop urgency, frequency, and faecal incontinence. Vaginal stenosis and premature ovarian failure can occur, but women should be advised to continue contraception until ovarian failure is proven. Male patients should be offered sperm banking to guard against temporary or permanent azoospermia.

9. **What are the prognostic factors in anal cancer and what is her estimated survival?**

In the absence of metastases, the size of primary tumour is the most useful predictor of survival, local control, and preservation of anorectal function. The 5-year overall survival is 75%, which is reduced by 20% in node-positive patients (i.e. to 55%). Overall survival is approximately 86% for T1–T2, 60% for T3, and 45% for T4 cancers. Anal margin cancers have a more favourable prognosis than those of the anal canal due to the decreased risk of nodal metastases. The median survival of patients with distant metastases is 9 to 12 months.

Since she has a T4N0 disease, her estimated 5-year survival is 45%.

10. **How will you assess response to treatment and how will you follow her up?**

A clinical assessment by physical examination is done 6–8 weeks after completion of treatment. Since squamous cell carcinomas regress slowly and continuously there is controversy regarding the optimal time to assess treatment response and plan salvage surgery. ACT II trial data showed that the complete clinical response (cCR) rate increased over time irrespective of the treatment arm: 60% of patients who did not achieve cCR at 11 weeks achieved it at 26 weeks. The cCR at 26 weeks correlated with PFS and OS. Thus, any decision of surgical salvage for persistent disease should be deferred until at least 26 weeks.

After cCR patients should to be followed up with DRE and inguinal examination every 3–6 months for 2 years and 6–12-monthly until 5 years, with the aim of detecting loco-regional recurrences or metastases and managing late effects of treatment proactively.

11. **If she were HIV positive how would you modify her treatment?**

Data from small series suggest that the outcome of HIV-positive patients is similar to that of HIV-negative patients. HAART (highly active antiretroviral therapy) needs to be started prior to commencing chemoradiotherapy. Radiotherapy and chemotherapy doses need to be modified due to the increased incidence of toxicities. Side-effects of radiotherapy can be more severe, with a dose of >30Gy necessitating diversion colostomy or APR in 6–12% of patients. Patients with haematological abnormalities or a previous history of significant opportunistic infections may not tolerate a full dose of mitomycin C and may require dose modification.

Further reading

Glynne-Jones R, Lim F. Anal cancer: an examination of radiotherapy strategies. *International Journal of Radiation Oncology Biology Physics* 2011; **79**: 1290–1301.

Kochhar R, Plumb AA, Carrington BM, Saunders M. Imaging of anal carcinoma. *American Journal of Roentgenology* 2012; **199**: W335–W344.

Lim F, Glynne-Jones R. Chemotherapy/chemoradiation in anal cancer: a systematic review. *Cancer Treatment Reviews* 2011; **37**: 520–532.

Uronis HE, and Bendell JC. Anal cancer: an overview. *The Oncologist* 2007; **12**: 524–534.

Case 15

Chromophobe renal cell carcinoma in an adult

Federica Recine and Cora Sternberg

Case history

A 32-year-old woman presented with left abdominal pain unresponsive to pain medications. An abdominal US revealed a left renal mass. CT scan confirmed a 9cm solid lesion in the upper pole of the left kidney with no evidence of metastatic disease (Fig. 15.1). Her past medical history was unremarkable and there was no family history of renal cancer.

She underwent a left laparoscopic radical nephrectomy and pathology revealed chromophobe renal cell carcinoma (ChRCC), Fuhrman grade 3, with focal involvement of the renal capsule. The surgical margins were negative and the adrenal gland was not infiltrated. A single hilar lymph node was found to be positive.

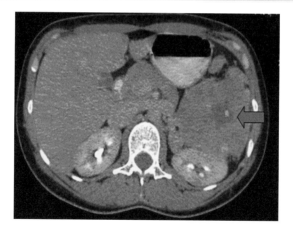

Fig. 15.1

Questions

1. What is the stage of her disease?
2. How do you assess her prognosis?
3. What specific features differentiate ChRCC from clear cell renal cell carcinoma (CCRCC)?
4. How do you follow up this woman?

Answers

1. What is the stage of her disease?

The stage is pT3a pN1 cM0 according to the AJCC. T3 is due to involvement of the Gerota fascia but not beyond it, and N1 due to regional node metastasis.

2. How do you assess her prognosis?

Two systems can be used to assess the risk of progression in localized RCC: the UCLA integrated staging system (UISS) and the stage, size, grade, and necrosis (SSIGN) score. The UISS provides prognostic prediction for localized and metastatic disease. UISS staging depends on the TNM classification, Furhrman grade, and ECOG performance status (Table 15.1). Based on the UISS, this patient has low-risk metastatic disease (N1M0) and has a predicted 5-year disease-specific survival of 32%.

Table 15.1 The UISS staging system

Patient group		Prognostic group			
		T stage	**Fuhrman grade**	**ECOG status**	**5-year disease-specific survival**
Localized disease (N0, M0)	Low risk	1	1–2	0	91.1%
	Intermediate risk	1	1–2	**1** or more	80.4%
		1	3–4	Any	
		2	Any	Any	
		3	1	Any	
		3	2–4	Any	
	High	3	2–4	**1** or more	54.7%
		4	Any	Any	
Metastatic disease	Low risk	N1M0	Any	Any	32%
		N2M0/M1	1–2	0	
	Intermediate risk	N2M0/M1	1–2	**1** or more	19.5%
			3	0, 1, or more	
			4	0	
	High	N2M0/M1	4	**1** or more	0%

3. What specific features differentiate ChRCC from clear cell renal cell carcinoma (CCRCC)?

RCC represents 85% of renal tumours and its incidence has significantly increased over the last 20 years. RCC is a heterogeneous disease including different histological types with various pathological and clinical characteristics. CCRCC is the most common form, accounting for 80% of RCC, while the remaining histological forms are grouped together as non-clear cell carcinoma, including ChRCC. ChRCC, which has an incidence of 6–11%, is an uncommon type of RCC with a better prognosis than other non-clear cell histologies. Because of the low incidence of this subtype of RCC and the limited number of cases in the literature the biology of this subtype of RCC and the therapeutic benefit from targeted therapies are not well understood, unlike for CCRCC.

ChRCC can be associated with overexpression of vascular endothelial growth factor (VEGF), a marker of angiogenesis that is crucial in tumour growth and metastases. Moreover, in this disease the *c-kit* (*CD177*) oncogene is upregulated, encoding a transmembrane tyrosine kinase receptor that plays a role in intracellular signal transduction.

The majority of cases of ChRCC are sporadic, but they may be associated with Birt–Hogg–Dubé (BHD) syndrome, an autosomal dominant hereditary cancer syndrome. Emerging data showing the pathogenetic mechanism in this hereditary form of ChRCC might suggest the molecular pathways driving the sporadic form of the disease. BHD syndrome is associated with germline inactivating mutations in the folliculin gene (*FLCN*) with a high risk of developing bilateral, multifocal ChRCC, skin lesions, and spontaneous pneumothorax.

FLCN is located on chromosome 17p11.2 and comprises 14 exons. The protein product of the *FLCN* gene, folliculin, is a tumour suppressor that is expressed in most tissues including the skin and its appendages, the lungs, and the kidney. Folliculin protein is a component of the cellular energy-sensing system and may interact with cellular-activated mitogen protein kinase (cAMPK) and mTOR pathways, suggesting a role also for mTOR antagonists in this disease.

4. How do you follow up this woman?

There is no standard protocol for follow-up for localized disease following surgery, but it often depends on the therapeutic possibilities upon recurrence. CT scan of the thorax and the abdomen is recommended for follow-up.

After surgery, there was no evidence of metastatic disease. She received immunotherapy with interferon-alpha (6 million IU) three times a week for 2 months at another oncology department. She was then followed closely and was free of disease for 7 months.

After 7 months she developed liver metastases in segments 3 and 8 (Fig. 15.2). She underwent surgical resection with a left hepatectomy and atypical resection of the eighth segment of the liver. The pathologist identified the presence of chromophobe cells, compatible with metastatic RCC. After this surgery, she was referred to our medical oncology department in Rome and observed with regular CT imaging.

Question

5. Is surgical resection of metastases recommended in ChRCC?

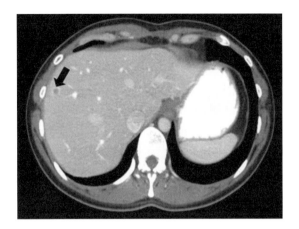

Fig. 15.2

Answer

5. Is surgical resection of metastases recommended in ChRCC?

Fewer than 5% of cases of ChRCC are metastatic at the time of diagnosis. Metastatic non-clear cell RCC has a poor survival, but the prognosis for patients with chromophobe tumours appears to be more favourable than for other subtypes of metastatic non-clear cell RCC. In fact, the median time to development of metastases from nephrectomy is twice as long for ChRCC as for other non-clear cell histologies.

While the most common site of renal cancer metastases is the lungs (75%), approximately 30–40% of patients will develop hepatic metastases. In most cases, liver metastases are multiple and occur in parallel with metastases to other sites.

Despite reports showing an improved survival with pulmonary metastatectomy in RCC, the role of liver-directed local treatments with surgery or radiofrequency ablation is not clearly established. Several clinical trials have shown that liver resection is effective and safe in the treatment of patients with hepatic metastases from RCC, even though these reports enrolled relatively small numbers of patients and did not distinguish between the different histological types. There are no established eligibility criteria for liver metastatectomy and the selection of patients is generally based on predicted prognosis and the feasibility of a margin-negative resection. Since patients with ChRCC seem to have a longer OS and DFS interval, those with resectable liver metastases are candidates for resection, which could be potentially curative even though this approach is still controversial in metastatic RCC.

Nine months after the second surgery, a routine CT scan revealed mediastinal lymph nodes, measuring 40, 21, and 24mm (Fig. 15.3). The patient declined a biopsy.

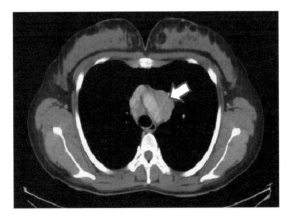

Fig. 15.3

Question

6. What therapy would you recommend?

Answer

6. What therapy would you recommend?

The treatment strategy for ChRCC is not well defined. The evidence of overexpression of VEGF and CD117 in ChRCC suggests a potential role for targeted therapies, but the reported data concerning the efficacy of TKIs in ChRCC are derived from retrospective analyses and expanded access trials.

The majority of clinical trials in metastatic RCC focus on patients with predominantly clear cell histology. The trial results rarely report differences in outcome between clear and non-clear cell types after TKI treatment, and therefore very little is known about the therapeutic benefit of TKIs in patients with non-clear cell RCC histology. However, the expanded-access trials of sunitinib and sorafenib included a considerable number of patients with non-clear cell histology and showed clinical efficacy of these agents in this type of RCC. Even though inhibitors of VEGF and mTOR pathways have been shown to have significant clinical benefit in advanced RCC, the role of these agents in patients with ChRCC remains unclear. Thus, the treatment options for this patient include sunitinib and sorafenib.

One month later she started therapy with sunitinib 50mg orally on a 4-week on, 2-week off schedule. After two cycles she obtained a partial response that was confirmed after an additional four cycles (Figure 15.4). She received a total of 16 cycles of sunitinib. She tolerated the therapy well and had no hypertension, but 1 year later she developed mild hypothyroidism.

Seven months later, she developed multiple metastases in segments 4, 6, and 8 of the liver.

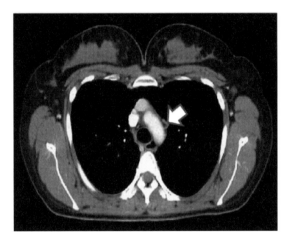

Fig. 15.4

Question

7.   Would you recommend another TKI for this patient with ChRCC?

Answer

7. Would you recommend another TKI for this patient with ChRCC?

The optimal sequential treatment in patients affected by advanced RCC is still under evaluation and there is no established sequence of therapy for clear cell or non-clear cell RCC.

Everolimus, a mTOR inhibitor, and axitinib, a VEGF-receptor TKI, are the two approved drugs in the second-line setting after TKI inhibitors for the treatment of metastatic RCC. However, several retrospective and prospective clinical trials have demonstrated the clinical benefit of the sequence of TKIs, showing that there is no cross-resistance among TKIs and VEGF inhibitors in RCC. Both sorafenib and suntinib applied in sequential treatment, after failure of previous anti-angiogenic therapy, have shown antitumor activity in advanced RCC. In the phase III AXIS trial (Rini et al. 2011), axitinib showed an advantage in PFS and equal OS compared with sorafenib in patients affected by metastatic clear cell RCC previously treated with sunitinib and cytokines. The retrospective trial published by Choueiri et al (2008) showed that in patients with advanced papillary and ChRCC, who were progressing with VEGF inhibitor therapy, a subsequent anti-VEGF therapy achieved stable disease. The INTORSECT trial, an open label randomized phase III trial, compared temsirolimus with sorafenib, in patients with RCC who had previous treatment with sunitinib (Hutson et al. 2012). This trial also included a proportion of patients with advanced non-clear cell RCC, and showed an improvement in overall survival of 4 months in the sorafenib arm, suggesting that temsirolimus was not superior to another TKI as a second-line treatment in patients who progressed on a previous TKI. These results suggest a potential role for the sequential treatment TKI–TKI; hence it is reasonable to recommend another TKI in this patient.

Treatment and follow up

The patient started treatment with sorafenib 800mg/day, which is ongoing at the time of writing.

Further reading

Beck SDW, Manish I, Patel IM, et al. Effect of papillary and chromophobe cell type on disease-free survival after nephrectomy for renal cell carcinoma. *Annals of Surgical Oncology* 2004; 11: 71–77.

Choueiri TK, Plantade A, Elson P, et al. Efficacy of sunitinib and sorafenib in metastatic papillary and chromophobe renal cell carcinoma. *Journal of Clinical Oncology* 2008; 26: 127–131.

Dudek AZ, Zolnierek J, Dham A, Lindgren BR, Szczylik C. Sequential therapy with sorafenib and sunitinib in renal cell carcinoma. *Cancer* 2009; 115: 61–67.

Hutson T, Escudier B, Esteban E, et al. Temsirolimus vs sorafenib as second line of therapy in metastatic renal cell carcinoma: results from the INTORSECT trial. ESMO Congress, Vienna, Austria, 28 September–2 October 2012. Abstract LBA 22. (Available at: http://abstracts.webges.com/viewing/view.php?congress=esmo2012&congress_id= 370&publication_id=918)

Larkin JM, Fisher RA, Pickering LM, et al. Chromophobe renal cell carcinoma with prolonged response to sequential sunitinib and everolimus. *Journal of Clinical Oncology* 2011; **29**: e241–e242.

Motzer RJ, Bacik J, Mariani T, Russo P, Mazumdar M, Reuter V. Treatment outcome and survival associated with metastatic renal cell carcinoma of non-clear-cell histology. *Journal of Clinical Oncology* 2002; **20**: 2376–2381.

Patard JJ, Leray E, Rioux-Leclercq N, et al. Prognostic value of histologic subtypes in renal cell carcinoma: a multicenter experience. *Journal of Clinical Oncology* 2005; **23**: 2763–2771.

Rini BI, Campbell SC, Escudier B. Renal cell carcinoma. *The Lancet* 2009; **373**: 1119–1132.

Rini BI, Escudier B, Tomczak P, et al. Comparative effectiveness of axitinib versus sorafenib in advanced renal cell carcinoma (AXIS): a randomised phase 3 trial. *The Lancet* 2011; **378**: 1931–1939.

Thelen A, Jonas S, Benckert C, et al. Liver resection for metastases from renal cell carcinoma. *World Journal of Surgery* 2007; **31**: 802–807.

Case 16

Prostate cancer

Jenny Nobes

Case history

A 65-year-old man presented to the colorectal surgical team with a 3-month history of progressive rectal pain and tenesmus. He had had no significant previous illnesses. Rectal examination revealed a hard, craggy, obstructing mass. Clinical examination was otherwise unremarkable. His ECOG performance status was 1. He was investigated with a CT scan of the abdomen and pelvis and MRI of the pelvis (Fig. 16.1).

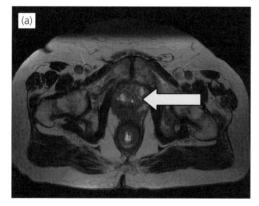

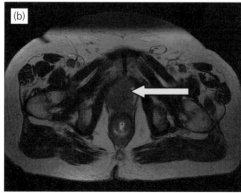

Fig. 16.1

Question

1. What does the MRI scan (Fig. 16.1) show?

Answer

1. What does the MRI scan (Fig. 16.1) show?

There is an extensive locally advanced prostatic tumour extending posteriorly to involve the anterior rectal wall and the external sphincter on the right. There is bone marrow heterogeneity in both inferior pubic rami, raising the possibility of metastases. The images provided do not demonstrate any enlarged lymph nodes.

Subsequently, he underwent a defunctioning colostomy and rectal biopsy. Histology showed a poorly differentiated carcinoma with no gland formation. Immunohistochemical staining demonstrated a diffuse strong membranous and paranuclear positivity with pancytokeratin with focal dot-like positivity, and diffuse cytoplasmic positivity with prostate-specific antigen (PSA). CD56, CD3, CD20, S100, chromogranin, TTF-1, CDX2, MyoD1, desmin, CK7, CK20, and CEA were negative.

Questions

2. How would you interpret the histology and how would you investigate further?
3. What would your initial treatment plan be?

Answers

2. How would you interpret the histology and how would you investigate further?

Immunohistochemistry suggests a poorly differentiated prostate carcinoma based upon PSA staining and both CK7 and CK20 negativity. A colorectal tumour is less likely because CEA and CK20 would be expected to be positive. Urothelial malignancies commonly stain with both CK7 and CK20.

He should have a serum PSA, FBC, and renal and bone biochemistry. To complete his skeletal staging an isotope bone scan is necessary, since he has already been shown to have possible bone metastases on MRI. It would be useful to also assess for deposits in his calvarium and appendicular skeleton with plain X-rays, given the high frequency of bone metastases with advanced prostate cancer.

3. What would your initial treatment plan be?

The mainstay of treatment for advanced prostate cancer is androgen deprivation therapy. This man is hormone-naïve. Therefore, he should initially be commenced on either luteinizing hormone releasing hormone (LHRH) analogues covered with anti-androgens to prevent testosterone flare, or a LHRH antagonist such as degarelix.

Palliative radiotherapy to alleviate his rectal pain should also be considered once testosterone suppression therapy is initiated. CT-guided virtual simulation would be required to encompass the pelvic soft tissue mass, treating to a dose such as 30Gy in 10 daily fractions over 2 weeks, given his good performance status.

Consideration should be given to a referral for specialist palliative care input given his new diagnosis of symptomatic advanced prostate cancer with the psychological impact of requiring a colostomy.

His serum PSA measured 483μg/L prior to commencement of androgen deprivation therapy with other blood parameters being in the normal range. The bone scan demonstrated abnormal increased tracer uptake within the skull, cervical, thoracic and lumbar spine, both scapulae, the right humerus, multiple ribs, pelvis, and both proximal femora. There was no other soft tissue disease demonstrated on CT.

After 3 months of hormonal therapy his PSA reached a nadir of 50μg/L, rising shortly thereafter to 150μg/ml despite the addition of an anti-androgen. Synchronously, he began to develop lower back pain with a bilateral radicular element. On examination he had full power in his lower limbs, normal reflexes, and no sensory deficit. His anal sphincter tone was preserved, and there was no perineal anaesthesia.

An urgent MRI (Fig. 16.2) of the whole spine was performed. CT staging revealed no visceral or nodal metastases. His ECOG performance status was 1.

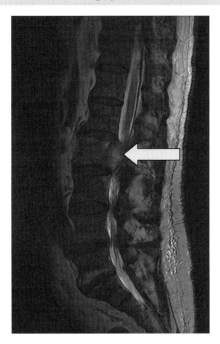

Fig. 16.2

Questions

4. What does the MRI scan (Fig. 16.2) show?
5. What would your initial management be based on these radiological findings?
6. Following this, what is your approach to systemically managing his prostate cancer, and what is the evidence base for this?
7. What are 'skeletal-related events' (SREs), and how would you reduce the risk of any further SREs?
8. What would you estimate his prognosis to be?
9. What would you advise him if he asks about prostate cancer screening for his sons?

Answers

4. What does the MRI scan (Fig. 16.2) show?

The MRI scan shows a large metastatic deposit involving the L2 vertebral body extending posteriorly into the central canal and compressing the cauda equina, with no cerebrospinal fluid around the nerve roots at this level.

5. What would your initial management be based on these radiological findings?

He should be commenced urgently on high-dose dexamethasone, e.g. 8mg twice daily, with a proton pump inhibitor for gastric protection. He has no neurological deficit so far from his cauda equina compression, has a good performance status, and has no extra-skeletal disease. His case should therefore be discussed with the spinal surgical team, and urgent spinal decompression and stabilization recommended to preserve his mobility.

Post-operatively, radiotherapy should be considered to the lumbar spine to reduce the risk of further neurological compromise at this level. A dose of 20Gy in five fractions would be one standard.

6. Following this, what is your approach to systemically managing his prostate cancer, and what is the evidence base for this?

Now that his prostate cancer has started to become hormone-refractory, he should be commenced on systemic chemotherapy with docetaxel 75mg/m^2 every 21 days for a maximum of 10 cycles, plus prednisolone 5mg twice daily. In 2004, the TAX 327 study reported a better survival with this regimen (18.9 versus 16.5 months) compared with mitoxantrone (Tannock et al. 2004). This regimen was therefore approved by NICE in 2006. An update of that study (Berthold et al. 2008) confirmed the significantly prolonged survival after 3-weekly docetaxel plus prednisolone than with mitoxantrone plus prednisolone (19.2 versus 16.3 months, $P = 0.004$).

Options for subsequent therapeutic lines would include abiraterone 1000mg daily until progression, or cabazitaxel 25mg/m^2 every 21 days for 10 cycles. A benefit in OS for both regimens has been reported in the COU-AA-301 and TROPIC trials, respectively (de Bono et al. 2010, 2011). The choice of regimen would depend on his performance status, bone marrow function, and previous response to taxane-based chemotherapy. At each stage, he should also be considered for entry into a clinical trial since there are several novel agents under investigation for advanced prostate carcinoma.

7. What are 'skeletal-related events' (SREs), and how would you reduce the risk of any further SREs?

SREs are defined as bone metastases resulting in pathological fracture, pain requiring radiotherapy to bone, surgery to bone, or malignant spinal cord compression. Radioactive strontium-89 and bisphosphonates such as intravenous pamidronate 90mg every 3–4 weeks are commonly prescribed in this clinical situation. However, the evidence for a delay in time to SRE and reduction in the number of SREs has only been demonstrated with intravenous zoledronic acid 4mg and the novel RANK ligand inhibitor denosumab, which is administered subcutaneously every 4 weeks.

This patient should therefore be considered for either zoledronic acid or denosumab in conjunction with his chemotherapy. Prior to commencement, he should undergo a baseline dental examination due to the approximate 10% risk of osteonecrosis of the jaw. He should also be prescribed oral calcium supplements to avoid the development of hypocalcaemia, providing that his serum-corrected calcium is not elevated.

8. What would you estimate his prognosis to be?

This depends in any individual on the response to further lines of systemic therapy. Based on the median survival advantages of taxane-based chemotherapy and abiraterone, an estimate of 12–24 months would be reasonable.

9. What would you advise him if he asks about prostate cancer screening for his sons?

The role of PSA screening has yet to be fully established. Large population-based screening studies in the United States and Scandinavia have reported a reduction in prostate cancer mortality, but with high numbers needed to screen before a life is saved. Nevertheless, in the UK, men over the age of 50, or over the age of 40 with a history of prostate cancer in a first-degree relative, are entitled to informed PSA testing. The risk of receiving a false negative or false positive result should be discussed, as should the options for management of early disease, including active surveillance.

Further reading

Berthold DR, Pond GR, Soban F, et al. Docetaxel plus prednisone or mitoxantrone plus prednisone for advanced prostate cancer: updated survival in the TAX 327 study. *Journal of Clinical Oncology* 2008; **26**: 242–245.

de Bono JS, Oudard S, Ozguroglu M, et al. Prednisone plus cabazitaxel or mitoxantrone for metastatic castration-resistant prostate cancer progressing after docetaxel treatment: a randomised open-label trial. *The Lancet* 2010; **376**: 1147–1154.

de Bono JS, Logothetis CJ, Molina A, et al. Abiraterone and increased survival in metastatic prostate cancer. *New England Journal of Medicine* 2011; **364**: 1995–2005.

Fizazi K, Scher HI, Molina A, et al. Abiraterone acetate for treatment of metastatic castration-resistant prostate cancer: final overall survival analysis of the COU-AA-301 randomised, double-blind, placebo-controlled phase 3 study. *Lancet Oncology* 2012; **13**: 983–992.

Ilic D, O'Connor D, Green S, Wilt TJ. Screening for prostate cancer: an updated Cochrane systematic review. *BJU International* 2011; **107**: 882–891.

Patchell RA, Tibbs PA, Regine WF, et al. Direct decompressive surgical resection in the treatment of spinal cord compression caused by metastatic cancer: a randomised trial. *The Lancet* 2005; **366**: 643–648.

Saad F, Gleason DM, Murray R, et al. A randomized, placebo-controlled trial of zoledronic acid in patients with hormone-refractory metastatic prostate carcinoma. *Journal of the National Cancer Institute* 2002; **94**: 1458–1468.

Smith MR, Saad F, Coleman R, et al. Denosumab and bone-metastasis-free survival in men with castration-resistant prostate cancer: results of a phase 3, randomised, placebo-controlled trial. *The Lancet* 2012; **379**: 39–46.

Tannock IF, de Wit R, Berry WR, et al. Docetaxel plus prednisone or mitoxantrone plus prednisone for advanced prostate cancer. *New England Journal of Medicine* 2004; **351**: 1502–1512.

Case 17

Testicular cancer

Susanna Alexander

Case history

A 66-year-old man presented to the emergency department with a 4-week history of increasing abdominal pain and fatigue. He was having conservative treatment for a diabetic foot ulcer under the vascular surgery team. He had lost 10kg in weight in the last 3 months. Clinical examination revealed an abdominal mass and palpable left supraclavicular lymphadenopathy. He had a CT scan of the chest and abdomen (Fig. 17.1). Biopsy from supraclavicular nodes showed a poorly differentiated neoplasm composed of monotonous sheets of pleomorphic large cells having abundant cytoplasm and hyperchromatic nuclei. The abnormal cellular population was strongly immunoreactive for placenta-like alkaline phosphatase (PLAP), OCT4, and CD117.

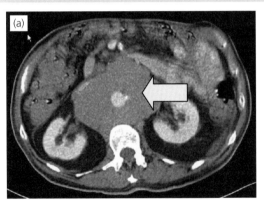 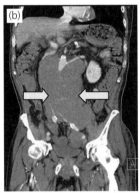

Fig. 17.1

Questions

1. What do the CT scans (Fig. 17.1) show?
2. How would you interpret the immunohistochemistry results?
3. What further investigations would you complete?

Answers

1. What do the CT scans (Fig. 17.1) show?

The CT scans show a large retroperitoneal mass surrounding the aorta (A). There is contiguous left common iliac and left external iliac lymphadenopathy (B). No other mass or destructive bone lesions were seen in the images. The differential diagnoses are lymphoma and germ cell tumour.

2. How would you interpret the immunohistochemistry results?

Immunohistochemistry shows this to be a seminoma. Seminoma is composed of a population of monotonous cells, and a very high proportion (98%) of seminomas show diffuse staining with antibodies to PLAP. Abnormal cells in testicular carcinoma *in situ* also stain with PLAP. CD117/c-KIT is specific for seminoma and positive in the majority of cases, but is rarely positive in embryonal carcinomas. OCT3/4 is a nuclear marker of classical seminoma and embryonal carcinoma. It has excellent sensitivity and specificity for these two tumours, and can be effectively used as the 'screen' for these neoplasms, especially when dealing with a metastatic tumour of unknown origin.

3. What further investigations would you complete?

A testicular ultrasound is needed to confirm the presence of a testicular mass even if there is clinically evident tumour. It will also assess the contralateral testis.

Serum tumour markers are prognostic factors when measured at diagnosis, and include beta human chorionic gonadotropin (β-hCG), α-fetoprotein (AFP), and lactate dehydrogenase (LDH). AFP and/or β-hCG are elevated in 80–85% of men with non-seminomatous germ cell tumours (NSGCTs). In contrast, serum β-hCG is elevated in fewer than 25% of seminomas, and AFP is not elevated in pure seminomas. LDH is elevated in 80% of patients with advanced testicular cancer and is important in deciding the prognostic group according to the International Germ Cell Cancer Collaborative Group (IGCCCG) classification (International Germ Cell Cancer Collaborative Group 1997). Tumour markers are also important in monitoring the response to treatment and detecting recurrence.

Testicular US showed a 1.6cm mass in the lower pole of the left testis which displayed course hypo-echogenicity and scattered microcalcification in keeping with a primary testicular tumour. The right testis was normal. The serum tumour markers were hCG 111IU/L (normal < 5IU/L), AFP < 1.0kU/L (normal 0–10kU/L), and LDH 931U/L (normal 125–243U/L).

Question

4. How would you treat this man?

Answer

4. How would you treat this man?

All patients with a testicular tumour should undergo an orchidectomy with division of the spermatic cord at the internal inguinal ring. In patients with disseminated disease and life-threatening pulmonary metastases, chemotherapy should be initiated immediately and orchidectomy delayed until clinical stabilization or completion of chemotherapy. In view of disseminated disease, this man should be considered for immediate chemotherapy.

Questions

5. If he needs chemotherapy, outline your pre-treatment assessment.
6. What is his estimated survival?

Answers

5. If he needs chemotherapy, outline your pre-treatment assessment.

Since this man has a metastatic germ cell tumour with good prognosis (seminoma with no non-pulmonary visceral metastases and normal AFP), the standard treatment option would be three cycles of BEP (bleomycin, etoposide, and cisplatin) chemotherapy. In patients for whom bleomycin is contraindicated or not advisable, four cycles of etoposide and cisplatin chemotherapy can be given instead. The MRC/EORTC TE20 study (de Wit et al. 2001) tested the equivalence of three versus four cycles of BEP and of the 5-day schedule versus 3 days per cycle in good-prognosis germ cell cancer. The study showed that three cycles of BEP with etoposide 500 mg/m^2 administered in 3 days was as effective as other regimens.

An alternative option in patients with significant comorbidities would be carboplatin chemotherapy given at area under the curve (AUC) 10 at 3-weekly intervals for a total of four cycles. This regimen was reported to be well tolerated, and 92% of patients were disease free in long-term (Oliver et al. 2004).

Pre-chemotherapy assessment includes the following:

◆ Record the WHO performance status, current height, weight, and body surface area.

◆ FBC, U&Es (including magnesium and calcium) and serum creatinine, liver function tests, AFP, HCG, and LDH.

◆ Consider formal measurement of creatinine clearance (creatinine clearance should ideally be >60ml/min) in patients with low surface area using either 24-hour urine collection or chromium-51 labelled ethylene diamine tetra-acetic acid (^{15}Cr-EDTA) measurement.

◆ Auditory assessment and pulmonary function tests including transfer factor.

◆ Informed consent.

◆ Where appropriate, discuss fertility issues and arrange sperm storage if necessary.

◆ Patients should have the support of a specialist nurse for holistic assessment.

6. What is his estimated survival?

The estimated 5-year PFS is 82% and the OS is 86% in patients with good-prognosis seminoma.

In view of his comorbidity, he proceeded with four cycles of AUC 10 carboplatin without initial orchidectomy. Re-staging showed normal serum markers and complete disappearance of the left supraclavicular node on CT scan. The post-chemotherapy abdominal CT scan is shown in Fig. 17.2.

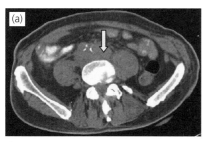
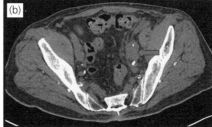

Fig. 17.2

Questions

7. What do the scans in Fig. 17.2 show?
8. What treatment would you recommend next?

Answers

7. What do the scans in Fig. 17.2 show?

The CT scan shows residual para-aortic and left pelvic lymphadenopathy.

8. What treatment would you recommend next?

He is advised to have an orchidectomy and is recommended to have a [18]FDG PET scan to confirm or refute active disease and therefore to decide between watchful waiting and active treatment.

Though there is no established role for [18]FDG PET in the staging of germ cell tumours or the re-staging of patients with non-seminomatous germ cell tumours after chemotherapy, it is recommended in patients with seminoma who have any residual disease at least 6 weeks after chemotherapy to identify active tumour. The SEMPET trial reported that [18]FDG PET correctly identified all cases of active tumour in residual lesions >3cm and 95% of active tumour in lesions of <3cm (specificity of 100% and sensitivity of 80%) (De Santis et al. 2004).

Histopathology after orchidectomy showed testis with extensive fibrous scarring and scattered chronic inflammatory cells, including pigment-laden macrophages, and atrophic seminiferous tubules suggesting post-chemotherapy scarring. The PET scan is shown in Fig. 17.3 (and in colour plate section).

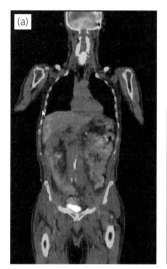
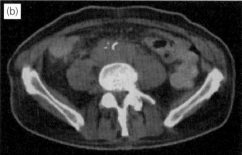

Fig. 17.3 (See also colour plate section)

Questions

9. What does the PET scan in Fig. 17.3 show?
10. What is the follow-up management?

Answers

9. What does the PET scan in Fig. 17.3 show?

The residual para-aortic and left pelvic adenopathy accumulates only background levels of ^{18}FDG, suggesting a metabolic complete response.

If PET scan is not available, repeat CT scan is advised at 2 and 4 months in patients with > 3cm residual tumour after chemotherapy for seminoma to ensure continuing regression of the mass.

10. What is the follow-up management?

The patient should have regular follow-up to detect treatable recurrent disease. The recommended minimum follow-up in metastatic testicular cancer includes 3-monthly physical examination, tumour marker estimation and chest X-ray, and 6-monthly abdomino-pelvic CT for 2 years, 6-monthly physical examination, tumour marker estimation, and chest X-ray for 3 years, and annual physical examination, tumour marker estimation, and chest X-ray thereafter.

Follow-up of this case

The patient continues to be well with no evidence of progression or recurrence 12 months after his orchidectomy.

Further reading

Albers P, Albrecht W, Algaba F, et al. EAU guidelines on testicular cancer: 2011 update. *European Urology* 2011; **60**: 304–319.

De Santis M, Becherer A, Bokemeyer C, et al. 2-18fluoro-deoxy-D-glucose positron emission tomography is a reliable predictor for viable tumor in postchemotherapy seminoma: an update of the prospective multicentric SEMPET trial. *Journal of Clinical Oncology* 2004; **22**: 1034–1039.

International Germ Cell Cancer Collaborative Group. International Germ Cell Consensus Classification: a prognostic factor-based staging system for metastatic germ cell cancers. *Journal of Clinical Oncology* 1997; **15**: 594–603.

Oliver RTD, Shamash J, Powles T, Somasundram U, Ell PJ. 20 year phase 1/2 study of single agent carboplatin in metastatic seminoma: could it have been accelerated by 72 hour PET scan response? *Journal of Clinical Oncology ASCO Meeting Proceedings* 2004; **22**: 4763 (abstract).

Sohaib AS, Koh W and Husband JE. The role of imaging in the diagnosis, staging and management of testicular cancer. *American Journal of Roentgenology* 2008; **191**: 387–395.

de Wit R, Roberts JT, Wilkinson PM, et al. Equivalence of three or four cycles of bleomycin, etoposide, and cisplatin chemotherapy and of a 3- or 5-day schedule in good-prognosis germ cell cancer: a randomized study of the European Organization for Research and Treatment of Cancer Genitourinary Tract Cancer Cooperative Group and the Medical Research Council. *Journal of Clinical Oncology* 2001; **19**: 1629–1640.

Case 18

Cervical cancer

Robert Wade

Case history

A 35-year-old woman presented to the gynaecology department with post-coital bleeding. At colposcopy she was found to have an exophytic tumour arising from her cervix. She underwent an EUA, staging MRI scan of the pelvis, and CT scans of the chest and the abdomen. The MRI showed a 4cm tumour centred on the cervix with parametrial extension (Fig. 18.1) with no evidence of nodal spread. Biopsy revealed a poorly differentiated squamous cell carcinoma. Blood tests showed a mild anaemia (haemoglobin 11.5g/dl, normal 13.0–17.0) but normal renal and liver function.

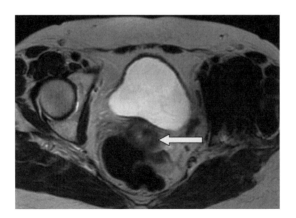

Fig. 18.1

Questions

1. What stage disease does this patient have?
2. Outline your treatment approach.

Answers

1. What stage disease does this patient have?

The patient has a FIGO (International Federation of Gynecology and Obstetrics) stage IIb TNM stage T2bN0M0 squamous cell carcinoma of the cervix. T1 disease is confined the cervix, T2 disease invades beyond the uterus but not to the pelvic side-wall or lower third of the vagina (T2a involves the upper two-thirds of the vagina; T2b involves parametria), T3 disease extends to the pelvic sidewall or lower third of the vagina and/or causes hydronephrosis (T3a involves the lower third of the vagina, T3b extends to the pelvic sidewall/causes hydronephrosis), and T4 disease involves mucosa of the rectum or the bladder or extends beyond the true pelvis.

2. Outline your treatment approach.

In stage IIB, stage III, and selected stage IV patients the standard treatment is chemoradiotherapy followed by brachytherapy. Concurrent cisplatin 40mg/m^2 once weekly for 5 weeks is given concomitantly with external beam radiotherapy Based on 13 trials, the addition of chemotherapy improved 5-year survival by 6% with an absolute improvement in PFS of 13% (Chemoradiotherapy for Cervical Cancer Meta-analysis Collaboration 2010).

At the MDT meeting treatment with chemoradiotherapy and brachytherapy is recommended.

Question

3. Describe your radiotherapy clinical target volume (CTV) and planning target volume (PTV) in detail. What dose would you prescribe?

Answer

3. **Describe your radiotherapy clinical target volume (CTV) and planning target volume (PTV) in detail. What dose would you prescribe?**

The structures that need to be treated with external beam radiotherapy include the primary tumour, vagina, uterus, parametria, pelvic sidewalls, and draining pelvic nodes. A contrast-enhanced planning CT with slice thickness ≤3mm should be performed. For node-negative disease the nodal CTV starts at the level of the junction of 4th and 5th lumbar vertebrae. The pelvic lymph nodes with a 7mm margin are outlined by following the course of the major pelvic arteries and veins. Taylor et al. (2005) and Small (2008) describe the appropriate structures that need to be included. The nodal CTV is grown a further 7mm to derive the nodal PTV. The uterus, parametria, cervix, and vagina are defined as the tumour CTV. A 15mm expansion of the tumour CTV to the PTV is required to ensure adequate tumour coverage. The nodal and tumour PTVs are then added together. The lower border of the treatment field tends to be at the level of the bottom of the obturator foramen or the inferior extent of vaginal involvement with a margin of 15mm. A dose of 45Gy in 25 fractions is prescribed to the International Commission on Radiation Units and Measurements (ICRU) reference point.

She is treated with 45Gy in 25 fractions with concomitant cisplatin.

Question

4. What clinical factors should be monitored during treatment?

Answer

4. What clinical factors should be monitored during treatment?

The main issues to watch out for apart from the direct side-effects of chemotherapy are haemoglobin levels and renal function. It is important to maintain haemoglobin levels above 12g/dl throughout treatment. A haemoglobin level below 12g/dl is recognized as a poor prognostic indicator and correction to 12g/dl may negate this factor. Overall treatment time is also important: the whole treatment from the start of external beam radiotherapy to the completion of brachytherapy should take no longer than 50 days, otherwise treatment becomes less effective. In the case of unexpected delays, Royal College of Radiologists guidelines for category 1 (patients with a tumour types for which there is evidence that prolongation of treatment affects outcome, and who are being treated with radical curative intent; see <https://www.rcr.ac.uk/docs/oncology/pdf/BFCO(08)6_Interruptions.pdf>) treatments should be followed. Two external beam fractions in a day with at least 6h between treatments need to be given to compensate for delays so that overall length of treatment stays within 50 days.

In the last week of external beam treatment the patient had a repeat MRI scan which showed a reduction in the size of her primary tumour. She underwent image-guided [high-dose-rate (HDR)] brachytherapy (IGBT) delivering four fractions of 7Gy each (over a period of 3 days with at least 6h between each fraction). She had a ring and tandem inserted in theatre but no interstitial needles were required. A MRI scan was performed with the applicator in situ.

Questions

5. Define high-risk CTV, intermediate-risk CTV, and point A.
6. What organs at risk (OARs) are important in IGBT and what are the accepted dose limits?
7. Which dosimetric parameters are important? How do you improve coverage to the high risk-CTV?
8. What outcome would you expect following treatment?

Answers

5. Define high-risk CTV, intermediate-risk CTV, and point A.

The principles behind IGBT are similar to those of external beam conformal planning. The basic technique requires placement of an intrauterine tube and ring in theatre under general anaesthetic with or without interstitial needles. In order to determine the optimal tandem/ring/needle combination the patient is anaesthetized and a ring and tandem are inserted, imaged, and planned prior to applicator removal. This allows the oncologist to determine whether interstitial needles are likely to be required, and their optimal placement. While CT localization is good enough to determine the OARs, a MRI scan is required to accurately define the high-risk CTV (HR-CTV) and to allow dose escalation. Ideally CT and MRI should be performed and fused on the treatment planning system. The HR-CTV includes residual tumour at the time of brachytherapy, the whole cervix, and any parametrial spread including gray zones (high-risk areas for micrometastatic disease which appear gray on T_2-weighted MRI sequences) and clinical findings from EUA. The location of the lower uterine arteries is helpful in defining the extent of the cervix. The intermediate-risk CTV (IR-CTV) reflects the extent of the tumour at initial presentation and takes into account tumour regression. In practice the IR-CTV is grown from the HR-CTV using a margin of between 5 and 15mm, editing out the OARs. The aim is to deliver four fractions of 7Gy each to the HR-CTV. Point A is the dose delivered to a point 2cm lateral to and 2cm superior to the cervical os. Figure 18.2 (see also colour plate section) shows the principal volumes of interest.

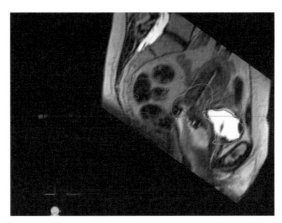

Fig. 18.2 (See also colour plate section)

6. What organs at risk (OARs) are important in IGBT and what are the accepted dose limits?

Four OARs are recognized—rectum, sigmoid colon, urinary bladder, and small bowel. The dose received by 2cm³ of an OAR is the dose-limiting constraint. The acceptable 2Gy equivalent doses (EQD2) by 2cm³ of OARs are: rectum 70–75Gy, sigmoid colon 70–75Gy, bladder 90–95Gy, and small bowel 70–75Gy. (Acceptable dose limits combine external beam and brachytherapy doses expressed as EQD2.)

7. Which dosimetric parameters are important? How do you improve coverage to the high-risk CTV?

The important dosimetric parameters are V100, D90, and EQD2 and physical dose to point A (V100 is the volume receiving 100% of the prescribed dose; D90 is the minimum dose delivered to 90% of the tumour target volume).

Optimization in IGBT is the process by which coverage to the HR-CTV is improved. With a ring and applicator the only way this can be done is by increasing the dwell times in the tandem, but this will increase toxicity to the anterior and posterior OARs. Interstitial needles allow the lateral dose to be increased without overdosing bladder, bowel, and rectum, thus improving tumour coverage and hopefully reducing morbidity. The dwell times in the intrauterine tube, ring, and interstitial needles can then be altered in order to maximize the D90 dose and the V100. A D90 of >75Gy to the HR-CTV according to the Royal College of Radiologists' guidance should achieve similar outcomes to historical series. Three-dimensional IGBT should achieve HR-CTVs of the order of 85–90Gy. Although in practice it is only really possible to optimize dose to one volume, a D90 of 60Gy to the IR-CTV should also be possible. Four fractions are delivered over 3 days with a minimum of 6h between each fraction with the applicator remaining *in situ* for all of that time.

8. What outcome would you expect following treatment?

Local control rates at 3 years from the Vienna group are 98% for tumours of 2–5cm and 92% for tumours >5cm (96% IIB; 86% IIIB). The expected 3-year cancer-specific survival is 83% for tumours of 2–5cm and 70% for tumours >5cm (84% IIB; 52% IIIB) (Potter et al. 2011). Other published series show similar results (e.g. Tan et al. 2009).

Further reading

Chemoradiotherapy for Cervical Cancer Meta-analysis Collaboration (CCCMAC). Reducing uncertainties about the effects of chemoradiotherapy for cervical cancer: individual patient data meta-analysis. *The Cochrane Database of Systematic Reviews* 2010; Jan 20 (1): CD008285.

Haie Meder C, Potter R, Van Limbergen E, et al. Recommendations from Gynaecological (GYN) GEC-ESTRO Working Group (I): concepts and terms in 3D image based 3D treatment planning in cervix cancer brachytherapy with emphasis on MRI assessment of GTV and CTV. *Radiotherapy and Oncology* 2005; **74**: 235–245.

Potter R, Haie Meder C, Van Limbergen E, et al. Recommendations from Gynaecological (GYN) GEC-ESTRO Working Group (II) concepts and terms in 3D image based treatment planning in cervix cancer brachytherapy—3D dose volume parameters and aspects of 3D image-based anatomy, radiation physics, radiobiology. *Radiotherapy and Oncology* 2006; **78**: 67–77.

Potter R, Georg P Dimopoulos JC, et al. Clinical outcome of protocol based image (MRI) guided adaptive brachytherapy combined with 3D conformal radiotherapy with or without chemotherapy in patients with locally advanced cervical cancer. *Radiotherapy and Oncology* 2011; **100/1**: 116–123.

Small W Jr, Mell LK, Anderson P, et al. Consensus guidelines for delineation of clinical target volume for intensity-modulated pelvic radiotherapy in postoperative treatment of endometrial and cervical cancer. *International Journal of Radiation Oncology Biology Physics* 2008; 71: 428–434.

Tan LT, Coles CE, Hart C, et al. Clinical impact of computerised tomography-based image-guided brachytherapy for cervix cancer using the tandem-ring applicator—the Addenbrooke's experience. *Clinical Oncology* 2009; **21**: 175–182.

The Royal College of Radiologists. *Implementing image guided brachytherapy for cervix cancer in the UK*. London: Royal College of Radiologists, 2009.

Taylor A, Rockall AG, Reznek RH, et al. Mapping pelvic lymph nodes: guidelines for delineation in intensity modulated radiotherapy. *International Journal of Radiation Oncology Biology Physics* 2005; **63**: 1604–1612.

Case 19

Ovarian cancer

Ioannis Gounaris and Christine Parkinson

Case history

A 47-year-old pre-menopausal woman presented with a few-week history of feeling excessively tired and unwell. She denied any abdominal symptoms and she had a past medical history of endometriosis and benign liver cysts. Clinical examination showed a palpable mass arising from the pelvis. Routine blood tests were normal. CA-125 was 54U/L (normal range 0–30). She underwent a CT scan of her abdomen and pelvis (Fig. 19.1).

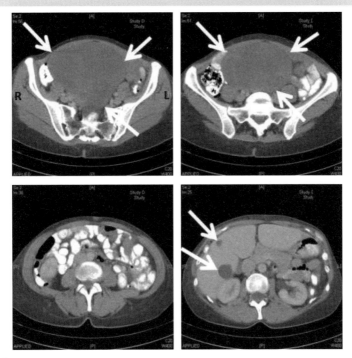

Fig. 19.1

Questions

1. What does the CT scan in Fig. 19.1 show?
2. Is the history of endometriosis relevant?
3. What is your next management decision?

Answers

1. What does the CT scan in Fig. 19.1 show?

The CT scan shows a large mass arising from the pelvis and extending into the abdomen. The mass appears complex, with cystic and solid components and septae (A, B). The ovaries cannot be seen separately from the mass. These features are suggestive of malignancy. Imaging does not show any peritoneal deposits (C). There are two hypodense lesions in the liver (D), and the larger one is well circumscribed while the smaller one has indistinct borders suspicious of a metastasis.

This patient had multiple prior CT and MRI scans of her liver to monitor her cystic disease, which confirmed the two lesions as cysts. If that had not been the case, further investigation with liver US and MRI scans would be warranted.

2. Is the history of endometriosis relevant?

Malignant transformation of endometriosis occurs in 0.5–1% of patients. However, this risk is restricted to specific histological subtypes, namely clear cell (CCC), endometrioid (EC), and low-grade serous (LGS) cancers. The odds ratios for these subtypes in women with self-reported endometriosis range between 2 and 3. There is no increased risk for the common ovarian cancer subtypes, high-grade serous (HGS), or mucinous and borderline tumours. In this patient, the history of endometriosis and the presence of a large pelvic mass with no upper abdominal spread make CCC or EC likely.

3. What is your next management decision?

The scans and the raised CA-125 are highly suggestive of malignancy. Therefore she should be reviewed by a gynaecological oncology surgeon, with the aim of undergoing a complete macroscopic removal of all tumour and comprehensive surgical staging, which includes total abdominal hysterectomy and bilateral salpingo-oophorectomy (TAH/BSO), infracolic omentectomy, peritoneal washings, and systematic peritoneal inspection and biopsies. The role of pelvic and retroperitoneal lymphadenectomy in women with normal-looking lymph nodes is debatable. When the decision is to proceed with primary surgery, pre-operative biopsy to confirm malignancy is not necessary.

For women staged initially with ultrasound, the risk of malignancy index (RMI), that takes into account ultrasound features, menopausal status, and CA-125 levels, can be calculated. A RMI score of >200 has a positive predictive value for malignancy of 80% with specificity of 89–92%.

At laparotomy, a large cystic mass arising from the right ovary was seen and removed. Unfortunately, the cyst ruptured during removal. There was no spread of the tumour beyond the ovary and no residual disease at the end of surgery. Histological examination revealed CCC of the right ovary (Fig. 19.2). Peritoneal biopsies were negative for malignancy. The final pathological staging was stage IC (rupture) clear cell ovarian cancer.

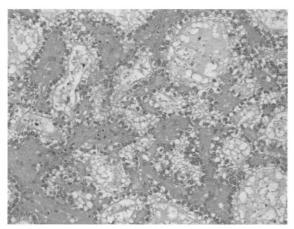

Fig. 19.2 (See also colour plate section)

Questions

4. What is the importance of histological subtypes in ovarian cancer?
5. What is your estimate of prognosis in this case?
6. Do you advise further treatment?
7. If you advise adjuvant chemotherapy, is there a preferred regimen?
8. Is there a role for radiotherapy in early stage CCC?

Answers

4. What is the importance of histological subtypes in ovarian cancer?

For many decades all epithelial ovarian cancers (EOCs) have been treated as a single disease entity. However, current understanding is that the five subtypes of EOC, namely HGS, CCC, EC, mucinous, and LGS, are distinct diseases. HGS cancers commonly present with advanced disease while most CCCs remain confined to the ovary at presentation and are surgically curable. CCC is characterized by increased incidence of thrombocytosis, hypercalcaemia, and venous thromboembolism, features that the clinician should keep in mind, especially during the perioperative period. CA-125 levels tend to be lower in CCC, a fact that can limit its utility in the diagnosis and monitoring of this disease. The effect of chemotherapy greatly differs between HGS and CCC tumours (see the answer to Question 6). Furthermore, whereas HGS cancers are molecularly characterized by ubiquitous TP53 mutations and frequent DNA repair defects (including *BRCA1/2* mutations), these features are exceedingly rare in CCC. The latter show predominantly mutations in the chromatin remodelling gene *ARID1A*, activating *PIK3CA* mutations, and almost universal overexpression of the transcription factor HNF1B. The absence of *BRCA1/2* mutations in CCC has obvious implications for the genetic counselling of these patients.

5. What is your estimate of prognosis in this case?

There has been considerable debate as to the prognosis of early stage CCC. In a series with contemporary pathology review from the British Columbia Cancer Agency (BCCA), patients with stage I–II CCC had better OS than patients with HGS (HR 0.55, 95% CI 0.37–0.79) (Anglesio et al. 2011). A meta-analysis of all published series again showed better OS for stage I–II CCC compared with HGS (HR 0.87, 95% CI 0.75–1.02) (Lee et al. 2011). Cyst rupture, either pre- or intraoperatively, has long been considered an adverse prognostic factor, and results in upstaging of stage IA/B disease to IC. However, at least three case series agree that, in CCC, cyst rupture does not influence prognosis; these patients have identical survival to stage IA patients (Hoskins et al. 2012). Therefore, the best estimate is that this patient's 5-year OS is around 90%, based on similar patients who underwent comprehensive surgical staging and received adjuvant chemotherapy.

6. Do you advise further treatment?

Adjuvant platinum-based chemotherapy is recommended for all but the lowest risk (stage IA/B, low grade) early stage EOC. This is based on the results of the ICON-1/ACTION combined analysis that showed an 8% 5-year OS advantage for platinum-based chemotherapy compared with observation (Trimbos et al. 2003). Paclitaxel is commonly added to carboplatin based on improved patient outcomes in studies that mostly enrolled patients with advanced HGS. Adjuvant chemotherapy with carboplatin and paclitaxel is recommended in all patients with CCC as this is considered a high-risk subtype. This recommendation is supported by the fact that the 130 patients with CCC enrolled in ICON-1/ACTION showed a similar benefit from chemotherapy to the whole trial population (albeit with wide confidence intervals). Nevertheless, there is extensive evidence from the advanced disease setting that CCC is comparatively resistant to chemotherapy. From the published case series, the median response to single-agent platinum and to a carboplatin–paclitaxel combination in advanced CCC is 20% and 40%, compared with >70% and >80%, respectively, in HGS. This fact, in addition to the excellent reported outcomes in stage IA/IC (rupture only) CCC, tempers enthusiasm for chemotherapy. It is not possible, at present, to be certain as to the exact contribution of chemotherapy to the reported 90% 5-year OS rate for these patients. It should be noted that two small case series from Japan, including 225 patients with stage IA/C CCC who received adjuvant chemotherapy and 67 who did not, failed to show any benefit from adjuvant chemotherapy (Takano et al. 2010, Takada et al.2012). To summarize, current best practice is to offer adjuvant chemotherapy to all patients with early stage CCC in the absence of contraindications. However, more clinical trials in this area are clearly required.

7. If you advise adjuvant chemotherapy, is there a preferred regimen?

The standard adjuvant chemotherapy for early stage CCC is carboplatin and paclitaxel (see answer to Question 6). However, the absolute survival benefit from chemotherapy is probably small, and therefore single-agent carboplatin is a reasonable choice in patients with comorbidities or those who wish to avoid the alopecia and peripheral neuropathy of taxane treatment. The combination of cisplatin and irinotecan is being compared with the standard carboplatin–paclitaxel doublet for the first-line treatment of CCC in an ongoing phase III study in Japan (JGOG 3017).

8. Is there a role for radiotherapy in early stage CCC?

Whole abdominal radiotherapy (WART) with a pelvic boost was used in the treatment of ovarian cancer in the 1960s and 1970s. However, it fell out of favour due to its long-term toxicities and the development of effective chemotherapy regimens. Adjuvant WART (22.5Gy to the pelvis in 10 fractions followed by 22.5Gy to the whole abdomen and pelvis in 22 fractions) has been a standard policy of the BCCA following surgery and adjuvant chemotherapy. In a recent report by this group the use of adjuvant radiotherapy was associated with a 20% absolute 5-year PFS advantage in high-risk (defined as stage IC (non-rupture)/II) CCC (Hoskins et al. 2012). A prospective trial is planned but, at present, there is no indication for the routine use of adjuvant radiotherapy in early stage CCC.

Treatment and follow-up

This patient received four cycles of adjuvant chemotherapy with carboplatin-paclitaxel cycles without any unexpected toxicities.

Further reading

Anglesio MS, Carey MS, Kobel M, et al. Clear cell carcinoma of the ovary: a report from the first Ovarian Clear Cell Symposium, June 24th, 2010. *Gynecologic Oncology* 2011; **121**: 407–415.

Hoskins PJ, Le N, Gilks B, et al. Low-stage ovarian clear cell carcinoma: population-based outcomes in British Columbia, Canada, with evidence for a survival benefit as a result of irradiation. *Journal of Clinical Oncology* 2012; **30**: 1656–1662.

Lee Y-Y, Kim T-J, Lim M-J, et al. Prognosis of ovarian clear cell carcinoma compared to other histological subtypes: a meta-analysis. *Gynecologic Oncology* 2011; **122**: 541–547.

Prat J. Ovarian carcinomas: five distinct diseases with different origins, genetic alterations, and clinicopathological features. *Virchows Archiv* 2012; **460**: 237–249.

Takada T, Iwase H, Iitsuka C, et al. Adjuvant chemotherapy for stage i clear cell carcinoma of the ovary: an analysis of fully staged patients. *International Journal of Gynecological Cancer* 2012; 22: 573–578.

Takano M, Sugiyama T, Yaegashi N, et al. Less impact of adjuvant chemotherapy for stage I clear cell carcinoma of the ovary: a retrospective Japan clear cell carcinoma study. *International Journal of Gynecological Cancer* 2010; **20**: 1506–1510.

Trimbos JB, Parmar M, Vergote I, et al. International Collaborative Ovarian Neoplasm Trial 1 and Adjuvant ChemoTherapy In Ovarian Neoplasm trial: two parallel randomized phase III trials of adjuvant chemotherapy in patients with early-stage ovarian carcinoma. *Journal of the National Cancer Institute* 2003; **95**: 105–112.

Case 20

Cancer in a renal transplant recipient

Christine Parkinson and Thankamma Ajithkumar

Case history

A 56-year-old woman presented with a 4-month history of bleeding per vagina. Her past medical history included end-stage renal failure for which she had had a cadaveric renal transplant 5 years previously, hypertension, and hypothyroidism. She was on azathioprine 75mg once daily, tacrolimus 3mg once daily, and prednisolone 1mg daily along with levothyroxine and pravastatin. She was having regular cervical cancer screening and the last smear 2 years ago was reported as normal.

A colposcopy showed a 3cm friable mass within the cervical canal extending through the external os. EUA showed a tumour extruding from the cervical os with no extension into the vagina or parametria. Biopsy showed a tumour composed of poorly differentiated adenocarcinoma with large polygonal cells having coarse chromatin and moderate cytoplasm. There were abundant mitoses (>10/10HPF). The cells stained strongly positive for cytokeratin 7, chromogranin, and synaptophysin, and were focally positive for p16 and CD56. The MRI scan is shown in Fig. 20.1.

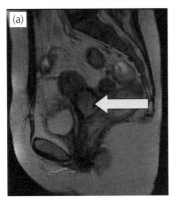 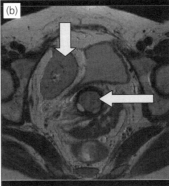

Fig. 20.1

Questions

1. What is your interpretation of the histopathology?
2. What does the MRI scan (Fig. 20.1) show?
3. Given the information available, what is the stage of the disease?
4. Discuss the challenges in her management.
5. What treatment would you offer?

Answers

1. What is your interpretation of the histopathology?

The histology shows a poorly differentiated adenocarcinoma with large cells having neuroendocrine features. Synaptophysin, chromogranin, and CD56 are neuroendocrine markers. Cytokeratin 7 is an epithelial marker, which together with CK20 can be used for the differentiation of epithelial neoplasms. The final diagnosis is a large cell neuroendocrine carcinoma, which usually shows >10 mitoses/10HPF. p16 is expressed in cervical carcinomas and dysplasias that are associated with high-risk HPV. Studies show that renal allograft recipients have an increased incidence of HPV-related malignancies.

2. What does the MRI scan (Fig. 20.1) show?

The MRI scan shows a bulky cervical mass (3cm × 2.7cm × 2.7cm) with marked distension of the rectum adjacent to the tumour (A, B). A normal non-hydronephrotic transplant kidney is seen in the right iliac fossa/right pelvis.

Other images confirmed the lack of parametrial invasion or involvement of the bladder or rectum. There was no enlargement of the pelvic or para-aortic lymph nodes. Small scarred kidneys were seen within the upper abdomen.

3. Given the information available, what is the stage of the disease?

Stage IB1—the tumour is limited to the cervix, and it is less than 4cm in diameter.

4. Discuss the challenges in her management.

Large cell neuroendocrine carcinoma (LCNEC) of the cervix is a rare and aggressive malignancy with poor prognosis even when treated in its early stage with multimodality treatment. Fewer than 80 cases have been reported since it was recognized as a separate entity in 1997. LCNEC has been reported to be associated with high-risk HPV types 16 and 18. The majority of patients present with early stage disease, and in spite of aggressive treatment >60% develop metastatic disease at first recurrence.

There is no consensus on the optimal management; treatment principles are adopted from the management of LCNEC of the lung. Chemotherapy is the main modality of treatment with the addition of radiotherapy and surgery. The commonly used chemotherapy regimens are cisplatin and etoposide, vincristine, doxorubicin, and cyclophosphamide, and carboplatin and paclitaxel. In spite of aggressive multimodality treatment, overall median survival is 15.5 months (0.5–151 months), with median survival being 19 months for stage I and 1.5 months for stage IV disease. Studies also show that earlier stage and addition of chemotherapy with platinum and etoposide improve survival.

In 2011 the Society of Gynaecological Oncology recommended the following treatment for neuroendocrine tumours of the gynaecological tract:

◆ Radical hysterectomy with lymphadenectomy followed by chemotherapy (cisplatin/etoposide) with or without radiotherapy for stage I–IIA disease of ≤4cm.

- Either chemoradiotherapy or neoadjuvant chemotherapy followed by surgery for stage I–IIA disease of >4cm.

- Chemoradiotherapy for advanced disease.

Some experts advise post-operative chemoradiotherapy for patients with stage I–IIA disease with the view of minimizing the risk of local recurrence; however, the exact benefit of such an approach is not known.

Prophylactic cranial irradiation in neuroendocrine tumours of the cervix is not advised as there is no proven benefit and the majority of patients die from disseminated distant metastases.

Malignancy is a well-recognized complication of transplantation. It can occur *de novo*, as a recurrence of a pre-existing malignancy, or from transmission of malignancy from the donor. However, there is no previous report of LCNEC in renal transplant recipients. The presence of a renal allograft poses the following challenges in the management of this patient:

- Though there is no contraindication for surgery, care should be taken to avoid damage to the new vasculature developed for the renal allograft.

- It is difficulty to deliver radiotherapy in view of the pelvic location of the renal allograft.

- There are challenges to the administration of chemotherapy, including an increased risk of graft loss due to direct cytogenetic effects or as a result of interactions with antirejection drugs and an increased risk of sepsis due to the additive or synergistic effects of chemotherapeutic and immunosuppressant drugs.

5. What treatment would you offer?

Since this patient has a stage IB1 neuroendocrine tumour of the cervix, the recommended treatment would be primary surgery with radical hysterectomy and lymphadenectomy followed by six courses of adjuvant chemotherapy using cisplatin and etoposide chemotherapy. Adjuvant pelvic radiotherapy is not advised in view of the pelvic renal allograft, even if there is any benefit.

A number of treatment modifications may be needed during her chemotherapy:

1. There is a risk of renal damage due to the nephrotoxicity of cisplatin. Hence renal function tests need to be carried out regularly and cisplatin should be administered with adequate hydration and diuresis (urine output >100ml/h).

2. There is a risk of infection due to the immunosuppressive effect of chemotherapy, and the immunosuppressants taken after transplant can also augment myelosuppression. Tacrolimuus and cyclosporine appear to have very minimal rates of neutropenia (<1%), whereas azathioprine, sirolimus, and mycophenolate mofetil have a slightly higher risk. Some experts substitute azathioprine with cyclosporine during chemotherapy; however, cyclosporine is contraindicated with cisplatin due to an enhanced nephrotoxicity, and therefore is not advised in this patient. Another reason why cyclosporine should be avoided in this patient is its potential interaction with etoposide, which decreases the excretion of cyclosporine and thereby increases its toxicity. Since it is difficult to estimate

the risk of febrile neutropenia in patients with organ transplants, it would seem prudent to use granulocyte colony-stimulating factor (G-CSF) prophylaxis and prophylactic antibiotics in transplant recipients.

3. Immunosuppressants may need to be modified after cancer treatment to keep immunosuppression to the minimum level needed to maintain graft-organ function. A change of immunosuppression to a regimen with an antiprolifera-tive effect, such as sirolimus or mycophenolate mofetil, might help to decrease the incidence of graft rejection and regress malignancy. However, the benefit of changing to an immunosuppressant with antiproliferative activity on the overall success of treatment is unknown. In renal transplant recipients, it is advised to reduce the tacrolimus concentration to a minimum and sirolimus is considered instead.

Progress and follow-up

In view of the stage IB1 disease, this patient underwent primary surgery involving radi-cal hysterectomy with lymphadenectomy. Prior to starting adjuvant chemotherapy, her immunosuppression was modified by stopping azathioprine and continuing on tacrolimus and prednisolone. Since she had a slightly raised serum creatinine, chemo-therapy was started with a 20% dose reduction of cisplatin and a 30% dose reduction of etoposide with G-CSF prophylaxis. After two cycles of chemotherapy the cisplatin dose was reduced by another 10% due to a deterioration in renal function. After completion of the chemotherapy, tacrolimus was changed to sirolimus based on its antiprolifera-tive effect. The patient remained well at the end of 5 years of follow-up.

Further reading

Ajithkumar TV, Parkinson CA, Butler A, Hatcher HM. Management of solid tumours in organ-transplant recipients. *Lancet Oncology* 2007; **8**: 921–932.

Embry JR, Kelly MG, Post MD, Spillman MA. Large cell neuroendocrine carcinoma of the cervix: prognostic factors and survival advantage with platinum chemotherapy. *Gynecologic Oncology* 2011; **120**: 444–448.

Gardner GJ, Reidy-Lagunes D, Gehrig PA. Neuroendocrine tumors of the gynecologic tract: a Society of Gynecologic Oncology (SGO) clinical document. *Gynecologic Oncology* 2011; **122**: 190.

Yoseph M, Chi M, Truskinovsky AM, et al. Large-cell neuroendocrine carcinoma of the cervix. *Rare Tumors* 2012; **4**: e18.

Case 21

Melanoma

Paul Nathan and Oliver Bassett

Case history

A 52-year-old white man presented to a plastic surgeon concerned about a mole on his back which had changed in pigmentation. He reported to be fit and well, had no signifi- cant past medical history, and took no medications. Examination was otherwise unre- markable. He underwent excision biopsy of the lesion and histopathology showed: 'a centrally situated area of nodular malignant melanoma 6mm in maximum diameter, and an area of adjacent radial growth phase component of superficial spreading type. It appears to have arisen from pre-existing melanocytic naevus. There is focal invasion into the reticular dermis (Breslow thickness 1.6mm). The overlying dermis is thin but not ulcerated. There is no evidence of vascular invasion. The minimum clearances in the lateral plane of section are 11mm (vertical) and 8mm (radial)'.

Questions

1. What is the patient's stage/prognosis and which feature not included in this pathology report can provide important prognostic information in thin melanomas?

2. Is further surgery recommended at this stage? What further procedure should be considered at this time?

Answers

1. What is this patient's stage/prognosis and which feature not included in this pathology report can provide important prognostic information in thin melanomas?

The AJCC published a revised staging system for cutaneous melanoma in 2009. The database used contained prospective data from more than 27,000 patients with stage I and II melanoma. Primary tumour (Breslow) thickness remained the most valuable independent prognostic indicator. Increasing tumour thickness (<1mm, >1mm, >2mm, and >4mm) showed a significant association with reduced 5- and 10-year survival rates. The presence of ulceration and mitotic rate were other important independent prognostic factors on multivariant analysis. Thin melanomas are rarely ulcerated; however, the presence of pathological ulceration in melanoma of any thickness upstages the tumour. The presence of one or more mitotic figure(s)/mm^2 in a thin melanoma (<1mm Breslow thickness) upstages the tumour from AJCC stage Ia to Ib with an associated reduction in the 10-year survival rate from 95% to 88% ($P < 0.0001$). The presence of ulceration or mitotic rate is now used to differentiate stage T1a and T1b. The level of invasion (Clark's level) is no longer used. The tumour under discussion was an AJCC stage IIa lesion with an associated 10-year survival of >80%.

2. Is further surgery recommended at this stage? What further procedure should be considered at this time?

The British Association of Dermatologists, the British Association of Plastic and Reconstructive and Aesthetic Surgeons, and the Melanoma Study Group UK published revised guidelines for the management of cutaneous melanoma in 2010 (Marsden et al. 2010). Surgery remains the only potentially curative treatment for primary melanoma. Current recommendations are for initial biopsy to be followed up with wide local excision to ensure removal of primary lesion and any local micrometastasis. A Cochrane Review (Sladden et al. 2011) showed that although there appeared to be a small survival advantage favouring wide excision it was not statistically significant, and current evidence is insufficient to define optimal excision margins. Current consensus is for lateral margins of 1cm for a tumour thickness of <1mm, 2cm for tumour thickness of >1mm, and 3cm for tumours >4mm. The guidance states that the final decision will be made depending on anatomical site, MDT discussion, and patient choice. Sentinel lymph node biopsy (SLNB) has become an established part of staging in melanomas >1mm thick of which approximately 20% will have a positive SLNB. The majority of patients with a positive node will go on to have completion lymphadenectomy, where 20% will show involved nodes in addition to the sentinel node.

Eight months after a normal clinical review the patient presented with discomfort in the right axilla. Examination revealed a palpable axillary mass of approximately 6cm × 7cm. CT scan confirmed a right axillary lymph node mass and the patient went on to have an axillary clearance which showed melanoma metastases in 29 out of 30 lymph nodes, including the apical node. There was evidence of extranodal spread and lymphovascular invasion. While awaiting adjuvant axillary radiotherapy the patient developed a palpable supraclavicular node.

Questions

3. Should further surgery be considered?
4. Is further imaging necessary?

Answers

3. Should further surgery be considered?

Despite limited evidence of survival benefit, the majority of clinicians would recommend metastatectomy in patients with oligometastatic disease. Early relapse, however, is a poor prognostic marker and heralds a high likelihood of the future appearance of further metastases. The majority of published data are from retrospective single-institution studies, which have a clear potential for selection bias. Morton (2007) presented results of a randomized phase III trial comparing an allogenic melanoma vaccine with a placebo in patients who had all undergone complete resection of metastasis to regional or distant sites. The study was stopped after an interim analysis due to no evidence of improved survival in the vaccine arm. However, the study showed an excellent survival for the whole study cohort, with 5-year survival of 42.3% in the stage IV patients. Sosman et al. (2011) published results of the Southwest Oncology Group trial which prospectively followed patients with stage IV disease who underwent complete resection. Four-year OS was 31%. It should be noted that all published studies were conducted before recent advances in treatment for metastatic melanoma when systemic therapeutic options were limited and response rates were notoriously poor. Simultaneously, PET/CT has become established in the assessment of metastatic spread in patients with melanoma prior to potential metastatectomy.

4. Is further imaging necessary?

This patient needs imaging with PET/CT prior to consideration for surgery.

The patient underwent a PET/CT scan prior to consideration for further surgery. This is shown in Fig. 21.1.

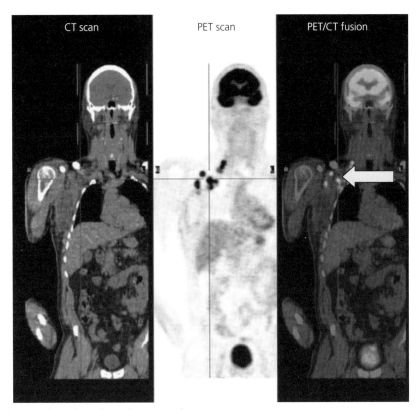

CT scan   PET scan   PET/CT fusion

Fig. 21.1 (See also colour plate section)

Question

5. What does the scan in Fig. 21.1 show?

Answer

5. What does the scan in Fig. 21.1 show?

The PET scan shows tracer uptake over the right axillary apical, infraclavicular, and supraclaviular lymph nodes.

The PET scan also shows unresectable loco-regional disease involving the skin and multiple regional lymph nodes as well as external iliac nodal disease.

Questions

6. What are the further treatment options?
7. What needs to be established before treatment options can be offered?

Answers

6. What are the further treatment options?

Further treatment options are systemic treatment using dacarbazine (DTIC; an alkylating agent), enrolment in an appropriate clinical trial, or vemurafenib (if *BRAF* mutation positive). Ipilimumab is a second-line treatment after chemotherapy.

Until recently the standard therapeutic agent available outside a clinical trial for metastatic melanoma was DTIC or its derivative temozolomide. In use since the 1970s, it has formed the mainstay of treatment for nearly 40 years. Published response rates are 5–15%, with the majority demonstrating only a short-lived partial response and no evidence of an increase in OS. Multiple trials comparing additional chemotherapy agents, immunotherapy, or biological modulating agents have shown no significant increase in survival when compared with DTIC alone.

Treatment options in metastatic melanoma have recently been revolutionized by the development of two new strategies now proven to increase OS. The first drug to be licensed was ipilimumab, a humanized monoclonal antibody that binds to an immune checkpoint molecule CTLA-4. Ipilimumab inhibits a negative regulatory pathway in T-lymphocyte activation, and therefore increases T-cell mediated immune killing. The first phase III trial recruited patients who had already progressed on therapy for systemic disease. They were randomly assigned to receive either a gp100 peptide vaccine, ipilimumab, or both treatments. Median OS in the ipilimumab treatment arms was 10.0 months compared with 6.4 in the gp100 vaccine arm. The most significant activity, however, appeared to be that a group of patients experienced durable long-term remission. Ipilimumab is given as a 3-weekly infusion, usually for a total of four doses. Grade 3 and 4 immune reactions occurred in 10–15% of patients, most commonly diarrhoea and skin reactions. Life-threatening colitis can occur and physicians should be particular vigilant for symptoms so prompt diagnosis can be made and steroid treatment commenced.

The second approach is with antagonists of oncogenic BRAF. Vemurafenib, an oral BRAF inhibitor, has been shown to increase OS in patients with stage IIIC and IV disease compared with DTIC. A phase III study (Chapman et al. 2011) showed a median PFS of 5.3 versus 1.6 months and OS at 6 months of 84% versus 64%. Several other similar drugs are currently in development and have shown promising early results.

7. What needs to be established before treatment options can be offered?

The *BRAF* mutation status needs to be established before deciding on further treatment.

Vemurafenib is a treatment option only in those patients whose tumours contain an acquired activating mutation in the *BRAF* oncogene. BRAF is a protein kinase which forms part of the RAS-RAS-MEK-ERK intracellular signalling pathway. The pathway is involved in cell proliferation, differentiation, and apoptosis. Approximately 50% of patients with melanoma will have a *BRAF* mutant tumour, of which the majority (90%) will be the single-point mutation V600E. Vemurafenib potently and specifically inhibits mutant BRAF, therefore the *BRAF* mutation status of a patient's tumour needs to be established before treatment options can be discussed. Mutation testing can be performed on the original tissue sample or on a biopsy of a metastatic lesion if the original sample is unavailable or insufficient. *BRAF* mutation testing should be considered in patients with high-risk primary melanoma and regional (stage III) disease and is the standard of care in stage IV disease. Treatment options for patients with wild-type (non-mutant) *BRAF* melanoma are still limited to chemotherapy or enrolment into a clinical trial.

The patient's tumour was found to be positive for the BRAF mutation and he entered into a clinical trial comparing DTIC with vemurafenib.

Question

8. How is vemurafenib administered and how should it be monitored?

Answer

8. How is vemurafenib administered and how should it be monitored?

Vemurafenib is administered in tablet form. The original study found a dose of 960mg twice daily to be the maximum tolerated dose. During the phase II trial 45% of patients required a dose reduction due to drug toxicities. Common side-effects include arthralgia, skin toxicity, and photosensitivity. Approximately 20% of patients develop skin lesions consistent with keratoacanthoma or squamous cell carcinoma thought to be due to signalling of braf/craf heterodimers in the presence of an upstream *ras* mutation. Therefore, regular skin examinations should be performed and surgical excision may be required. Patients should be advised to wear high-factor sun protection because severe sunburn can occur even in cloudy conditions. Median time to confirmed radiological response in the phase III trial was 1.45 months; however, a clinical improvement can be seen in as little as 2 weeks, and the drug can rapidly palliate patients suffering severe tumour-related symptoms.

Treatment and follow-up

The patient was initially randomized to DTIC within the clinical trial but showed progression of disease after 14 weeks. He crossed over to the vemurafenib arm where he has shown an ongoing prolonged response to treatment lasting >18 months.

Further reading

Balch CM, Morton DL, Gershenwald JE, et al. Sentinel node biopsy and standard of care for melanoma. *Journal of the American Academy of Dermatology* 2009; **60**: 872–875.

Chapman PB, Hauschild A, Robert C, et al. Improved survival with vemurafenib in melanoma with BRAF V600E mutation. *New England Journal of Medicine* 2011; **364**: 2507–2516.

Eigentler TK, Caroli UM, Radny P, Garbe C. Palliative therapy of disseminated malignant melanoma: a systematic review of 41 randomised clinical trials. *Lancet Oncology* 2003; **4**: 748–759.

Hodi FS, O'Day SJ, McDermott DF, et al. Improved survival with ipilimumab in patients with metastatic melanoma. *New England Journal of Medicine* 2010; **363**: 711–723.

Marsden JR, Newton-Bishop JA, Burrows L, et al. Revised UK guidelines for the management of cutaneous melanoma 2010. *Journal of Plastic, Reconstructive and Aesthetic Surgery* 2010; **63**: 1401–1419.

Morton DL, Mozzillo N, Thompson JF, et al. An international, randomized, phase III trial of bacillus Calmette–Guerin (BGC) plus allogenic melanoma vaccine or placebo after complete resection of melanoma metastatic to regional or distant sites. *Journal of Clinical Oncology* 2007; **25** (18s): abstract 8508.

Sladden MJ, Balch C, Barzilai DA, et al. Surgical excision margins for primary cutaneous melanoma: a summarised Cochrane review. *Clinical and Experimental Dermatology* 2011; **36**: 334–335.

Sosman JA, Moon J, Tuthill RJ, et al. A phase 2 trial of complete resection for stage IV melanoma: results of Southwest Oncology Group Clinical Trial S9430. *Cancer* 2011; **117**: 4740–4746.

Sosman JA, Kim KB, Schuchter L, et al. Survival in BRAF V600–mutant advanced melanoma treated with vemurafenib. *New England Journal of Medicine* 2012; **366**: 707–714.

Case 22

Merkel cell carcinoma

Thankamma Ajithkumar

Case history

An 80-year-old woman presented with a rapidly growing lesion on her left cheek. She had first noticed this lesion 8 months previously, and it was slowly growing until her presentation. She underwent excision of the lesion, and the histopathology showed a 2.5cm infiltrating tumour mass composed of monomorphic small round blue cells with little visible cytoplasm. Numerous mitotic figures were seen, and the cells stained positive for CD20 and negative for TTF-1 and CD7.

Question

1. What is your diagnosis?

Answer

1. What is your diagnosis?

The combination of CD20 positivity and TTF-1 negativity suggests that the tumour is a Merkel cell carcinoma (MCC). MCC is a neuroendocrine tumour of the skin, characterized by a perinuclear punctuate or dot-like pattern of CD20 staining. Differential diagnosis of a small round cell neoplasm of the skin includes metastatic small cell lung cancer (SCLC), MCC, lymphoma, and melanoma. The use of a selective panel of immunohistochemistry tests helps to make a definitive diagnosis (Table 22.1).

Table 22.1 Immunohistochemistry in small round cell neoplasms of the skin

Tumour	CK20	CK7	TTF-1	LCA	S100
MCC	+	−	−	−	−
SCLC	−	+	+	−	−
Lymphoma	−	−	−	+	−
Melanoma	−	−	−	−	+

LCA, leucocyte common antigen.

Shortly after the initial excision, the lesion recurred; she therefore underwent further surgery which showed similar cancer with invasion of deep muscles and a close excision margin.

When she attended the oncology clinic 4 months later, she had developed another nodule of 1.5cm near the edge of the previous skin graft.

Question

2. How would you proceed?

Answer

2. How would you proceed?

Further evaluation requires a detailed history including significant comorbidities and a clinical examination to delineate the local disease and identify any enlarged regional nodes. Since MCC has a high risk of both regional nodal and distant metastasis, she needs staging with CT/MRI of the head and neck and a CT scan of the chest and abdomen. Some authorities also recommend [18]FDG-PET scan in patients with regional nodal metastases. The role of ^{68}Ga-DOTATOC PET is being investigated.

CT staging showed no regional nodal disease or metastatic disease.

Questions

3. Outline your further management.
4. Should you consider systemic treatment for her, and if so why?
5. What is the role of primary radiotherapy in MCC?

Answers

3. Outline your further management.

She is recommended to have radical radiotherapy to the loco-regional area. Without radiotherapy, after wide excision of tumour, >40% patients develop local recurrence and >80% develop regional recurrence (this woman had two successive local recurrences within a short period of time). Therefore adjuvant radiotherapy to a dose of 50–56Gy is recommended.

Optimal management of clinically node negative disease is uncertain. Studies show that the risk of nodal disease correlates with size of the primary tumour. Patients with a primary tumour of >1cm have a >30% risk of nodal involvement. Sentinel node biopsy is helpful in deciding the need for regional nodal treatment. Patients with negative sentinel node biopsy do not need any nodal treatment, whereas those with positive nodes are treated with radical radiotherapy or complete nodal dissection, followed by adjuvant nodal radiotherapy if there is extracapsular extension or advanced nodal disease. Patients who have not had a sentinel node biopsy or lymphadenectomy are recommended to have regional nodal radiotherapy to a dose of 45–50Gy.

This patient is recommended to have radiotherapy to the primary tumour, parotid bed, and ipsilateral cervical nodes (because of unknown nodal status).

4. Would you advise adjuvant chemotherapy for her?

The benefit of adjuvant chemotherapy in MCC is controversial and therefore not advised outside clinical trial settings.

5. What is the role of primary radiotherapy in MCC?

Primary radiotherapy is an acceptable option when surgery is not technically feasible or the patient is medically unfit for surgery. A dose of ≥60Gy is recommended and gives a 75% in-field control rate.

She received 60Gy in 30 fractions to left side of the cheek, left parotid, and upper neck and 50Gy in 25 fractions to the left lower neck. One year after completion of radiotherapy she presented with two subcutaneous nodules over the anterior chest wall just above the costal margin. Excision showed MCC. Her ECOG performance status was 0. Figure 22.1 shows the re-staging CT scans.

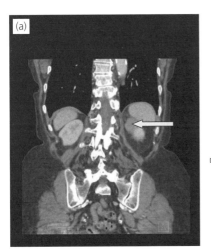
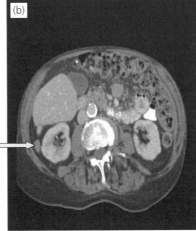

Fig. 22.1

Questions

6. What does the imaging in Fig. 22.1 show?
7. What is your management at this stage?
8. What is her prognosis?

Answers

6. What does the imaging in Fig. 22.1 show?

There is a soft-tissue mass (3.2cm) between the upper pole of the left kidney and the diaphragm (A). Another mass is seen posterior to the right lobe of the liver (1.4cm) (B). The scan also showed a pancreatic lesion and multiple lung and pleural nodules (not shown here).

7. What is your management at this stage?

Combination chemotherapy is the standard treatment for distant metastatic disease. Radiotherapy has a role in symptom relief. Patients with a solitary metastasis may be considered for surgery, though there is a paucity of evidence concerning this approach.

Because of the similarities between MCC and SCLC the chemotherapeutic approach is same as that for SCLC. The regimen of cisplatin/etoposide yields a response rate of 60% with a 36% complete response in MCC whereas cyclophosphamide, doxorubicin, and vincristine (CAV) produces a 70% response rate with a complete response of 35%. The average duration of response is 8 months. Complete responders may have a better duration of response (20 months) than those with a partial response (3 months).

8. What is her prognosis?

Median survival of patients with metastatic MCC is 8–12 months, with a 5-year survival of 25%.

After four courses of a carboplatin/etoposide regimen, she achieved a complete radiological response. Six months later she presented with right shoulder pain, and a re-staging CT scan was done (Fig. 22.2).

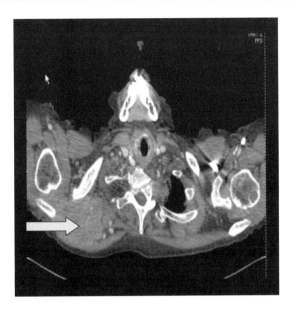

Fig. 22.2

Questions

9. What does the scan in Fig. 22.2 show?

10. What is your management now?

Answers

9. What does the scan in Fig. 22.2 show?

The CT scan shows a soft tissue mass arising posterior to the right glenoid, extending into the posterior chest.

10. What is your management now?

Since she has pain from the locally advanced tumour, she might benefit from palliative radiotherapy. The radiotherapy dose ranges from 8–10Gy as one fraction to 20–30Gy in five to ten fractions.

If her ECOG performance status remains good (0–1), she may be offered further systemic treatment. Despite a high initial response rate, relapses are frequent after platinum/etoposide for MCC and SCLC. Patients are classified as sensitive to treatment if recurrence occurs ≥90 days after the end of first-line treatment or resistant if disease recurs within 90 days. Patients who progress during first-line treatment are classified as refractory. Sensitive patients may be re-challenged with first-line treatment, though there are no randomized trial data regarding this approach. Topotecan is the only approved second-line treatment independent of time of progression, and results in an OS 84 days longer than the best supportive care.

Progress and follow-up

She was re-challenged with carboplatin/etoposide for four courses, which yielded only a partial response. She died 3 months later, 33 months after her first presentation.

Further reading

Becker JC. Merkel cell carcinoma. *Annals of Oncology* 2010; **21**(Suppl 7): vii81–vii85.

Gonzalez RJ, Padhya TA, Cherpelis BS, et al. The surgical management of primary and metastatic Merkel cell carcinoma. *Current Problems in Cancer* 2010; **34**: 77–96.

Kudchadkar R, Deconti R. Systemic treatments for Merkel cell carcinoma. *Current Problems in Cancer* 2010; **34**: 97–107.

Rao NG. Review of the role of radiation therapy in the management of Merkel cell carcinoma. *Current Problems in Cancer* 2010; **34**: 108–117.

Schrama D, Ugurel S, Becker JC. Merkel cell carcinoma: recent insights and new treatment options. *Current Opinion in Oncology* 2012; **24**: 141–149.

Case 23

Soft tissue sarcoma

Helen Hatcher

Case history

A 21-year-old man presented to the emergency department with a painful, swollen right foot. He remembered falling over a kerb after drinking alcohol a few weeks previously and had associated the swelling with this. He had no significant medical history prior to this. He had an X-ray and MRI of the right foot (Figs 23.1 and 23.2). A biopsy showed tumour cells arranged in small and large nests surrounded by thin fibrovascular stroma lined by small round blue cells (resembling lymphoma). The structure showed an alveolar growth pattern in small sections of the tumour. Occasional multinucleated giant cells were seen alongside rhabdomyoblasts with small areas of necrosis. Immunohistochemistry showed no staining for CD20, CD45, or HMB45, mild staining for pancytokeratins, and positivity for actin, desmin, and MyoD1.

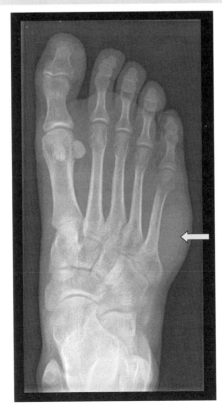

Fig. 23.1

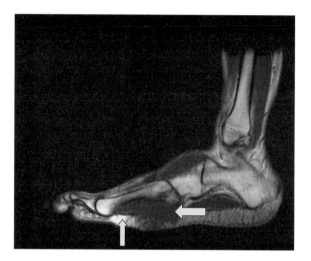

Fig, 23.2

Questions

1. What do the X-ray (Fig. 23.1) and MRI (Fig. 23.2) show?
2. What does the biopsy indicate?
3. What further tests are needed on the tissue?
4. What further investigations should you do?

Answers

1. What do the X-ray (Fig. 23.1) and MRI (Fig. 23.2) show?

The X-ray shows a soft tissue swelling associated with the fifth metatarsal but no evidence of fracture or bony involvement at that point. The MRI shows the soft tissue lesion between the metatarsal and the skin. There is enhancement of the subcutaneous tissue suggesting involvement of the overlying skin and structure.

2. What does the biopsy indicate?

The biopsy findings are highly suggestive of an aggressive soft tissue sarcoma; immunohistochemistry is suggestive of an alveolar rhabdomyosarcoma (ARMS). Rhabdomyosarcoma is a rare sarcoma of striated muscle with an annual incidence of 1 in 1,000,000. It is the most common childhood soft tissue sarcoma and has a peak incidence in teenagers and young adults. It tends to occur in skeletal structures and can occur anywhere in the body, but common sites include the limbs, the paratesticular region, and the head and neck. It most often presents as a painless lump, often quite rapidly growing, but it can cause pain if it is close to certain structures, for example in the head and neck where compression of adjacent structures can occur. The histological subgroups of rhabdomyosarcoma include embryonal (ERMS; more common in those under 16), alveolar, and pleomorphic (which tends to occur in those over 30). ARMS accounts for approximately 20–30% of all rhabdomyosarcomas. Metastatic disease at diagnosis occurs in 25–30% of patients. The most frequent sites of metastatic spread include the lymph nodes, bone, and bone marrow.

Tumour cells in ARMS are relatively small with scant cytoplasm. They have round regular nuclei with a monotonous chromatin pattern. The cells form aggregates interrupted by fibrovascular septae, and within these aggregates areas of discohesion often form, resulting in spaces that resemble the alveoli of the lung. In some ARMS cases there are few fibrovascular septae, no alveoli-like spaces, and a predominant cellular small round cell population; the term 'solid variant' applies to this situation.

In addition to general immunohistochemical markers to identify rhabdomyosarcoma, certain markers aid in the identification of ARMS. Immunostaining for myogenin and MyoD shows different patterns between ARMS and ERMS, such that most cells within an ARMS tumour stain positive whereas fewer cells within an ERMS tumour do so. In addition, based on microarray studies that distinguish fusion-positive ARMS from fusion-negative ERMS, AP2β and p-cadherin were found to be specific markers for the fusion-positive ARMS subtype.

3. What further tests are needed on the tissue?

Further information should be gained by genetic studies using either polymerase chain reaction (PCR) or FISH to look for specific gene rearrangements. ARMS is associated with specific gene rearrangements which give prognostic information. The most common is the *PAX3/FOXO1* fusion gene followed by *PAX7/FOXO1* (Box 23.1). These fusion genes encode fusion transcription factors with a *PAX3* or *PAX7* DNA-binding domain and *FOXO1* transactivation domain. Among ARMS tumours, approximately 60% are *PAX3/FOXO1*-positive, 20% are *PAX7/FOXO1*-positive, and 20% are fusion negative (Fig. 23.3).

Box 23.1 Molecular cytogenetics in ARMS

- t(2;13)(q35;q14)—*PAX3/FOXO1* in 60–85%
- t(1;13)(p36;q14)—*PAX7/FOXO1* in 15–20%
- N-myc amplification in 50%

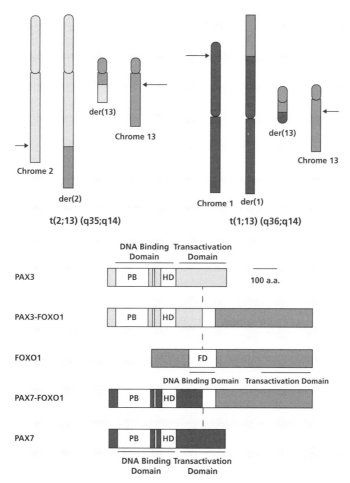

Fig. 23.3 Diagram to show the comparison of wild-type and fusion products associated with the t(2;13) and t(1;13) translocations. The paired box (PB), octapeptide, homeobox (HD), and fork head domain (FD) are indicated as open boxes, and transcriptional domains (DNA-binding domain, DBD; transcriptional activation domain) are shown as solid bars. The vertical dashed line indicates the translocation fusion point.

Reprinted from Atlas Genet Cytogenet Oncol Haematol January 2009; Barr FG. Soft tissue tumors: Alveolar rhabdomyosarcoma <http://atlasgeneticsoncology.org/Tumors/AlvRhabdomyosarcID5194.html> by permission of the Atlas.

The *PAX7/FOXO1* fusion is often amplified in tumours (70% of *PAX7/FOXO1*-positive cases) whereas the *PAX3/FOXO1* gene fusion is much less frequently amplified in tumours (5% of *PAX3/FOXO1*-positive cases). Gene amplification appears to be one mechanism for increasing the expression level of the gene fusion in ARMS tumour cells.

4. What further investigations should you do?

He needs further investigation with a CT chest, abdomen, and pelvis, bone scan, and bone marrow examination. Patients with disease at sites at risk of meningeal involvement (e.g. a parameningeal primary) also need an examination of the cerebrospinal fluid.

The CT scan is shown in Fig. 23.4 There was no other disease elsewhere.

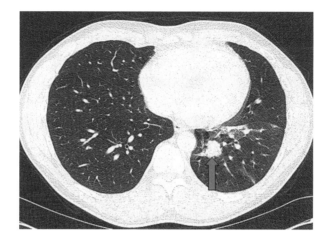

Fig. 23.4

Questions

5. What does the CT scan in Fig. 23.4 show?
6. What treatment should he be offered?
7. What are the prognostic factors in ARMS?

Answers

5. What does the CT scan in Fig. 23.4 show?

The CT scan shows a mass close to the left lower lobe bronchus with interstitial shadowing. It indicates metastatic disease to the lungs which places this patient in the high-risk group.

6. What treatment should he be offered?

The optimal treatment involves intensive chemotherapy (in high-risk cases the commonly used regimen is IVADo—ifosfamide, vincristine, actinomycin D, and doxorubicin) followed by radiotherapy and/or surgery tailored to the individual sites of disease and the prognostic group. For localized disease, surgery should be undertaken ideally after four or five cycles of chemotherapy. Radiotherapy is used for high-risk tumours (large, alveolar histology), in cases where surgery is not possible, or in the palliative setting. The tumours are extremely radio- and chemosensitive and an excellent response is often seen to initial chemotherapy but with (in ARMS) a high risk of breakthrough disease or recurrence soon after the completion of treatment. An Italian study has suggested the benefit of a maintenance treatment with 12 cycles of oral cyclophosphamide and intravenous vinorelbine (Casanova et al. 2004), and at the time of writing this is being tested in a European rhabdomyosarcoma trial. At relapse, a number of regimens are used but there is no consensus on the best one. Examples include regimens containing cyclophosphamide/topotecan, irinotecan/temozolamide, or ifosfamide. A phase II European relapse trial is randomizing between vincristine/irinotecan or vincristine/irinotecan/temozolamide (<http://clinicaltrials.gov/ct2/show/NCT01355445>).

7. What are the prognostic factors in ARMS?

Patients with ARMS tumours have a poorer outcome than patients with ERMS tumours. The 4-year failure-free survival rates for patients with localized and metastatic ARMS are 65% and 15%, respectively. Other risk factors that influence the outcome of ARMS include primary site, size of the primary tumour, extent of local spread, and the presence of nodal and distal metastases.

In an analysis of patients from the IRS-IV study, patients with localized *PAX3/FOXO1*- and *PAX7/FOXO1*-positive ARMS had comparable outcomes (Sorensen et al. 2002). In contrast, among patients presenting with metastatic disease, those with *PAX3/FOXO1*-positive tumours had a significantly poorer outcome than those with *PAX7/FOXO1*-positive tumours (4-year OS of 8% compared with 75%, $P = 0.0015$).

Further reading

Barr FG. Gene fusions involving PAX and FOX family members in alveolar rhabdomyosarcoma. *Oncogene* 2001; **20**: 5736–5746.

Casanova M, Ferrari A, Bisogno G, et al. Vinorelbine and low-dose cyclophosphamide in the treatment of pediatric sarcomas: pilot study for the upcoming European Rhabdomyosarcoma Protocol. *Cancer* 2004; **101**: 1664–1671.

Ferrari A, Dileo P, Casanova M, et al. Rhabdomyosarcoma in adults. A retrospective analysis of 171 patients treated at a single institution. *Cancer* 2003; **98**: 571–580.

Gerber NK, Wexler LH, Singer S, et al. Adult rhabdomyosarcoma survival improved with treatment on multimodality protocols. *International Journal of Radiation Oncology Biology Physics* 2013; **86**: 58–63.

Missiaglia E, Williamson D, Chisholm J, et al. PAX3/FOX01 fusion gene status is the key prognostic molecular marker in rhabdomyosarcoma and significantly improves current risk stratification. *Journal of Clinical Oncology* 2012; **30**: 1670–1677.

Sorensen PH, Lynch JC, Qualman SJ, et al. PAX3-FKHR and PAX7-FKHR gene fusions are prognostic indicators in alveolar rhabdomyosarcoma: a report from the children's oncology group. *Journal of Clinical Oncology* 2002; **20**: 2672–2679.

Sultan I, Qaddoumi I, Yaser S, et al. Comparing adult and pediatric rhabdomyosarcoma in the surveillance, epidemiology and end results program, 1973 to 2005: an analysis of 2,600 patients. *Journal of Clinical Oncology* 2009; **27**: 3391–3397.

Case 24

Bone sarcoma

Helen Hatcher

Case history

A 19-year-old woman presented with a fracture of the left femur (Fig. 24.1), sustained after a football tackle during a summer camp overseas. The femur was pinned, but because of abnormalities seen during surgery, samples of bone were sent for histopathological examination, which confirmed a diagnosis of osteosarcoma.

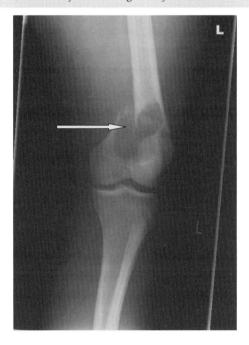

Fig. 24.1

Questions

1. What is the relevance of the fracture, and what impact does it have on the prognosis of osteosarcoma?
2. What further investigations are recommended?
3. What treatment should be recommended next?
4. What is the role of radiotherapy in this case?

Answers

1. What is the relevance of the fracture, and what impact does it have on the prognosis of osteosarcoma?

Pathological fracture in osteosarcoma is associated with a worse prognosis, especially if the lesion is pinned, due to potential dissemination of tumour along the bone marrow and into the blood stream. In one study, osteosarcoma patients with pathological fracture had lower 10-year overall survival than those without (34% versus 58%, $P < 0.01$) (Bramer et al. 2007).

2. What further investigations are recommended?

Staging and investigations at diagnosis include MRI of the primary and the joints on either side to examine the extent of disease and to detect skip lesions. CT of the chest is needed to exclude lung metastases and bone scan to rule out bone metastases. Investigations which will be required prior to starting systemic treatment include echocardiogram, nuclear medicine evaluation of renal function (GFR), FBC, biochemistry, coagulation screen, and placement of a central venous catheter to administer chemotherapy.

Staging in this patient confirmed that the left femur was the only site of disease.

3. What treatment should be recommended next?

Ideally, the pathological fracture should not have been pinned but stabilized by brace, case, or external fixation following a biopsy. Chemotherapy is the primary treatment in patients with pathological fracture, followed by limb-salvage surgery if possible.

Since this patient had a pinning of the pathological fracture, which carries a high risk of disseminated micrometastases, the priority at this stage is to give systemic treatment with combination chemotherapy. There is no worldwide consensus on the standard chemotherapy. The current UK recommendation is a combination of cisplatin given with doxorubicin and high-dose methotrexate (the MAP regimen). A recent meta-analysis showed that the MAP regimen gives a significantly better outcome than a combination of cisplatin and adriamycin (Anninga et al. 2011).

The abnormal bone should be resected after two cycles of MAP, preferably with an endoprosthetic replacement. (The EURAMOS trial (<http://www.ctu.mrc.ac.uk/euramos/euramos_i_trial.asp>) has been set up to evaluate the role of changing chemotherapy if a poor response is seen at the time of surgery and to evaluate the benefit of the addition of biological agents such as interferon, but has completed recruitment.) Outside a trial, four more cycles of MAP are given post-operatively. In patients over the age of 40, high-dose methotrexate is unlikely to be safely tolerated so these patients are treated with cisplatin and doxorubicin alone. There is controversial evidence about the use of another biological agent, mifamurtide (a liposomal formulation of the immune stimulant muramyl tripeptide phosphatidylethanolamine), which can be given postoperatively with MAP chemotherapy. In selected cases, it can improve 6-year overall survival by an additional 8% (78%

versus 70%). This is licensed for the treatment in resectable osteosarcoma, and the evidence should therefore be discussed with the patient.

4. What is the role of radiotherapy in this case?

Radiotherapy is not routinely given in osteosarcoma as this is a relatively radiore-sistant disease. However, in selected cases, such as pathological fracture, tumour crossing the cortex, and poor margins at surgery, radiotherapy may be given to improve local control.

She completed treatment and went onto regular follow-up with chest X-ray and X-ray of the left femur every 3 months. The chest X-ray taken 9 months after completion of treatment is shown in Fig. 24.2.

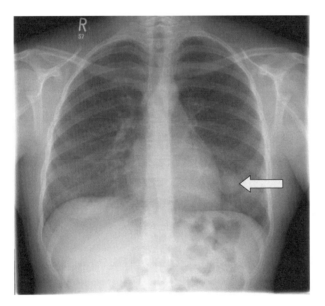

Fig. 24.2

Questions

5. What does the chest X-ray in Fig. 24.2 show?
6. How do you investigate?
7. What are the treatment options and what is the role of chemotherapy?
8. What is the prognosis?

Answers

5. What does the chest X-ray in Fig. 24.2 show?

The chest X-ray shows a solitary round lesion in the left chest close to the heart border. Given the relatively short time since completion of treatment for osteosarcoma, this is likely to represent a lung metastasis.

6. How do you investigate?

A CT scan of the chest should be done to rule out multiple metastases and define in more detail the lesion seen on the chest X-ray. A bone scan should also be done to rule out bone metastases. The CT scan showed a single lesion in the left lower lobe (Fig. 24.3).

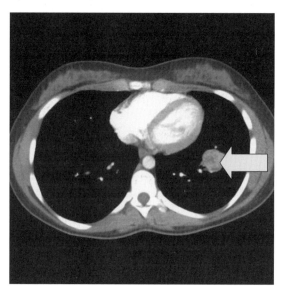

Fig. 24.3

7. What are the treatment options and what is the role of chemotherapy?

The treatment options include removal of the metastasis by wedge resection or lobectomy and further chemotherapy. Ideally, surgery, which removes the lesion with a safe margin but with the lowest impact on lung function (wedge resection), should be performed if possible. There are no randomized trials examining the role of chemotherapy before or after surgery. However, relapse in a site that had no previous lung nodule within less than a year is a poor prognostic sign and many clinicians would advocate chemotherapy with a drug that is known to be active in osteosarcoma and that was not used in the neoadjuvant or adjuvant setting. In this situation, ifosfamide with etoposide or high-dose ifosfamide may be considered. This can be given pre- and post-operatively—giving some pre-operatively allows for systemic treatment upfront without a post-operative delay if the recovery period is prolonged.

8. What is the prognosis?

In this specific patient the prognosis is guarded because relapse has occurred within less than a year, but long-term survival is still possible in 10–15% of patients. Factors which predict for a poorer outcome in this situation include the short time between the end of treatment and relapse, suggesting a rapidly growing tumour.

After further treatment, the patient remained well for 23 months but was found to have an abnormal chest X-ray at follow-up. CT staging is shown in Fig. 24.4.

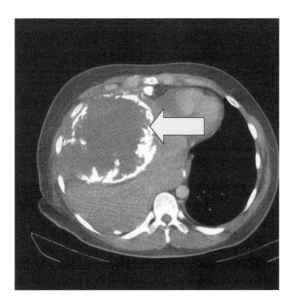

Fig. 24.4

Question

9. What options does she have now and what is her prognosis?

Answer

9. What options does she have now and what is her prognosis?

The CT scan (Fig. 24.4) shows an extensive lesion with calcification. In view of the large size of the recurrence there is no realistic curative treatment option. Palliative options, if the patient chooses to opt for palliative chemotherapy, could include gemcitabine with docetaxel or oral etoposide. Opting for supportive care only would also be an option if the patient chooses. Her prognosis is now severely limited due to the rapid occurrence (between 3-monthly chest X-rays) of a large tumour bulk. Palliative care services should be involved from an early stage.

Further reading

Anninga JK, Gelderblom H, Fiocco M, et al. Chemotherapeutic adjuvant treatment for osteosarcoma: where do we stand? *European Journal of Cancer* 2011; **47**: 2431–2445.

Bramer JA, Abudu AA, Grimer RJ, Carter SR, Tillman RM. Do pathological fractures influence survival and local recurrence rate in bony sarcomas? *European Journal of Cancer* 2007; **43**: 1944–1951.

DeLaney TF, Park L, Goldberg SI, et al. Radiotherapy for local control of osteosarcoma. *International Journal of Radiation Oncology Biology Physics* 2005; **61**: 492–498.

Meyers PA, Schwartz CL, Krailo MD, et al. Osteosarcoma: the addition of muramyl tripeptide to chemotherapy improves overall survival-a report from the Children's Oncology Group. *Journal of Clinical Oncology* 2008; **26**: 633–638.

Brain tumour

Thankamma Ajithkumar

Case history

A 33-year-old woman presented with nausea and a tingling sensation over her left hand for 2 weeks, and one episode of grand mal seizure. She had a CT scan followed by MRI of the brain (Fig. 25.1). A CT scan of the chest, abdomen, and pelvis and blood tests were unremarkable. Her ECOG performance status was 1.

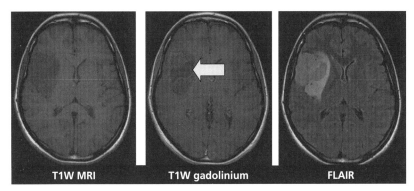

Fig. 25.1

Questions

1. What do the scans in Fig. 25.1 show?
2. Outline your initial management.

Answers

1. What do the scans in Fig. 25.1 show?

T_1-weighted MRI shows an irregular hypo-intense mass in the right temporoparietal region, which enhances peripherally on administration of gadolinium. The FLAIR (fluid-attenuated inversion recovery) image shows a hyper-intense lesion representing the tumour and surrounding oedema. There is minimal pressure effect on the anterior horn of the right lateral ventricle. The appearance is suggestive of an aggressive intrinsic brain tumour, and since it is a single lesion with normal staging investigations it is most likely to be a high-grade glioma.

2. Outline your initial management.

The initial management includes general medical measures and referral to a MDT meeting for discussion of primary surgical management. Steroid and antiepileptic drugs (AEDs) are important in the initial management of patients with suspected brain tumours. Steroids help to reduce the intracranial pressure and reverse symptoms. Steroids are started at the maximum dose likely to reverse symptoms and rapidly titrated against the patient's symptoms. The usual agent used is dexamethasone 2–16mg daily. The temptation to treat seizures with a steroid, except as a short-term expedient, should be avoided.

All patients with brain tumour-associated seizure should be treated with AEDs. However, there is no established role for the prophylactic use of AEDs in patients with brain tumours.

Long-acting carbamazepine is probably the best initial drug, starting at 100mg twice daily and increasing after 2 weeks to 200mg twice daily if necessary, after the estimation of blood levels of the drug. Lamotrigine and sodium valproate are effective alternatives in patients who tolerate carbamazepine poorly. Phenytoin has the convenience of once daily administration, with a starting dose of 200mg followed by a blood level assessment 7–10 days later. If seizures continue to be a problem after optimal monotherapy, levetiracetam 250mg twice daily is added, and the dose increased according to response and tolerance to a maximum of 1.5g twice daily.

Many AEDs are enzyme inducers and hence non-enzyme inducing (or weak enzyme inducing) drugs are preferred for patients with brain tumours in whom chemotherapy or biological therapies are considered (see Table 25.1).

Pain management is according to the WHO analgesic ladder. Depression, a common problem in patients with brain tumours, needs to be appropriately managed.

Table 25.1 Recommended AEDs for brain tumour-associated seizures

Type of seizure	Recommended AED
Infrequent, focal	Lamotrigine 25mg once daily for 2 weeks and then increased to 50mg once daily. Increase by a maximum 100mg every 1–2 weeks. As monotherapy the maximum dose is 100–200 mg daily OR Levetiracetam 250mg once daily and increased after 1–2 weeks to 250mg twice daily; further increase in steps of 250mg twice daily every 2 weeks to a maximum of 1.5g twice daily AND clobazam 10–20mg once daily if needed
Frequent, focal (at least once daily) Generalized	Levetiracetam 500mg twice daily increasing to 1000mg twice daily within a week AND clobazam 10–20mg once daily
Generalized, presenting as severe clusters or status epilepticus	Treat as status epilepticus and once stabilized convert to levetiracetam or lamotrigine

She was started on levetiracetam 250mg twice daily and dexamethasone 8mg daily. She underwent an 'awake' craniotomy and excision of the tumour. The histopathology showed an anaplastic oligodendroglioma with frequent mitoses and microvascular proliferation, but without necrosis or microcalcification. The MIB-1 index was 50%.

Questions

3. What is the advantage of an 'awake' craniotomy?
4. What is the significance of the MIB-1 index?
5. What further management would you recommend?
6. What are the prognostic factors and what is the estimated prognosis?

Answers

3. What is the advantage of an 'awake' craniotomy?

Surgical techniques for brain tumours are constantly evolving. Patients with a suspected brain tumour will usually have an intraoperative frozen section or smear prior to attempting a full resection. Studies suggest that there is a correlation between the extent of resection and median survival in high-grade gliomas. Gross tumour resection (no post-operative contrast enhancement) results in a better median survival than subtotal resection (post-operative nodular enhancement) in both anaplastic astrocytoma (58 versus 34 months) and glioblastoma (13 versus 8 months). Therefore a complete or maximal surgical resection with minimal injury to neighbouring critical structures is the aim of surgery. Cortical mapping during 'awake' craniotomy is useful in the resection of tumours inside, or adjacent to, functional brain areas. Intraoperative stimulation of cortical and subcortical areas and related tracts allows one to identify and mark active areas, and facilitates sparing of functional areas during resection. In 'awake' craniotomy, the initial craniotomy and preliminary stimulation are done with the patient asleep. After arousal, sedative/hypnotic anaesthesia allows the patient to respond to motor and language commands but still provides subsequent amnesia.

4. What is the significance of the MIB-1 index?

The MIB-1 index (a marker of proliferation) is a predictor of survival in astrocytic tumours. In diffuse astrocytoma (grade 2), the MIB-1 index is usually less than 4% (mean 2.5%). The MIB-1 index of anaplastic astrocytoma (grade 3) is in the range of 5–10% and that of glioblastoma (GBM; grade 4) in the range of 15–20%. The survival of grade III tumours with a MIB-1 index of >15–20% is similar to that of glioblastoma.

5. What further management would you recommend?

The current standard treatment for glioblastoma is concomitant chemoradiotherapy followed by adjuvant temozolomide. A phase III trial has shown that the addition of concomitant and adjuvant temozolomide to radical radiotherapy in patients with glioblastoma improves survival compared with radiotherapy alone (a 5-year survival 10% versus 2% and median survival of 14.6 versus 12.1 months). A subset analysis has shown that patients with methylguanine methyl transferase (MGMT) methylated tumours have the best survival advantage with the addition of temozolomide to radiotherapy (median survival 23 versus 15 months). However, the role of concomitant chemoradiation in grade 3 tumours is yet to be proved, and the standard post-operative treatment in grade 3 tumours is radiotherapy alone.

It has been recognized that the presence of necrosis in oligodendroglial tumours is associated with a poor prognosis and therefore 'anaplastic oligodendrogliomas with necrosis' are classified as glioblastoma. There might be a subset of patients with anaplastic oligodendroglioma without necrosis but with a high MIB-1 index (>15%) with an outcome equivalent to glioblastoma. Some authorities recommend treatment of these tumours similarly to glioblastoma with concomitant/adjuvant temozolomide.

Thus, in view of the high MIB-1 index, this patient is recommended to have radical radiotherapy with concomitant/adjuvant temozolomide.

6. What are the prognostic factors and what is the estimated prognosis?

The median survival of anaplastic oligodendroglioma after radical treatment is 4.5 years. The presence of necrosis is associated with a poorer median survival (35 months), whilst the presence of the 1p/19q code deletion is associated with a better median survival (8.5 years with deletion and 3.7 years with no deletion). Other good prognostic factors include isocitrate dehydrogenase (IDH1) mutation and MGMT methylation.

The median survival of patients with typical anaplastic oligodendroglioma is 4.5 years; however, in the presence of a very high MIB-1 index it is likely that the prognosis may be similar to glioblastoma (12–16 months).

The patient completed radical radiotherapy and six courses of adjuvant temozolomide. A repeat MRI scan showed no evidence of contrast enhancement to suggest recurrent disease.

Five months later she presented with pain radiating to the right leg and an abnormal sensation in the right leg but without impaired mobility. The gadolinium-enhanced MRI scan is shown in Fig. 25.2.

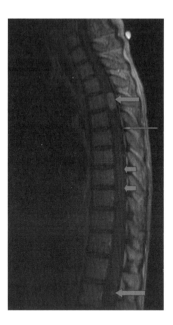

Fig. 25.2

Questions

7. What does the MRI scan in Fig. 25.2 show?
8. What is your immediate management?

Answers

7. What does the MRI scan in Fig. 25.2 show?

MRI shows a contrast-enhancing intradural mass at the thoracic level (the mass measures 2.3cm and is at the level of T4). There are two other nodules, one at the level of T5/6 and another at the level of L1. There is some subtle linear contrast enhancement of the cord surface. Other images show cord compression and cord oedema. This appearance is consistent with drop metastases with leptomeningeal disease.

Symptomatic leptomeningeal or intramedullary metastasis can occur in up to 2% of patients with high-grade gliomas. It is common in infratentorial tumours. The mechanisms of dissemination include spread by invasion of the choroid plexus, through subpial, perivascular, and subarachnoid spaces, and via the cerebrospinal fluid. The common sites of drop metastases are the lower thoracic and lumbosacral regions. The clinical features include radicular pain and sensory and motor deficits suggesting cord compression or cauda equina syndrome. Surgical decompression is not an option for the majority of patients due to the diffuse nature of the disease; however, it may be useful in selected patients with a discrete mass causing cord compression and to achieve better pain control. Radiotherapy is useful in relieving pain temporarily, but seldom improves the neurological deficit. There is no proven role for systemic and/or intrathecal chemotherapy. Prognosis is poor with a median survival of 2–4 months.

8. What is your immediate management?

High-dose dexamethasone (16mg daily) and neurosurgical review for decompression of the thoracic lesion is the initial management. If surgery is not appropriate, emergency radiotherapy is indicated.

The patient underwent decompressive surgery. The pathology was consistent with a primary neuroectodermal tumour, suggesting an aggressive transformation of oligo-dendroglioma. Although she received thoracic spinal radiotherapy to a dose of 20Gy in five fractions her mobility continued to deteriorate. A MRI scan done 2 months later is shown in Fig. 25.3.

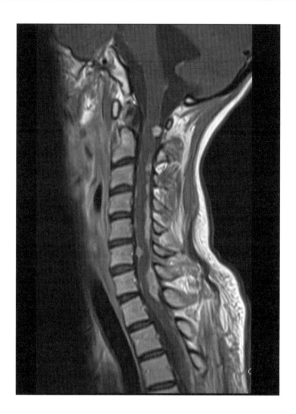

Fig. 25.3

Questions

9. What does the MRI scan in Fig. 25.3 show?
10. What is your management?

Answers

9. What does the MRI scan in Fig. 25.3 show?

The MRI shows progressive leptomeningeal/intradural contrast-enhancing disease involving the whole of area of the spinal canal.

10. What is your management?

She has rapidly progressive disease, and her treatment is essentially symptomatic and palliative. The patient died 4 weeks after the last scan.

Further reading

Brat DJ, Prayson RA, Ryken TC, Olson JJ. Diagnosis of malignant glioma: role of neuropathology. *Journal of Neurooncology* 2008; **89**: 287–311.

Burnet NG, Lynch AG, Jefferies SJ, et al. High grade glioma: imaging combined with pathological grade defines management and predicts prognosis. *Radiotherapy Oncology* 2007: **85**: 371–378.

Ricard D, Idbaih A, Ducray F, et al. Primary brain tumours in adults. *The Lancet* 2012; **26**: 1984–1996.

Scoccianti S, Detti B, Meattini I, et al. Symptomatic leptomeningeal and intramedullary metastases from intracranial glioblastoma multiforme: a case report. *Tumori* 2008; **94**: 877–881.

Case 26

Hodgkin lymphoma

Isabella Maund and Michael Williams

Case history

A 25-year-old woman presented with a painless lump on the left side of her neck. She was otherwise well. Biopsy performed under ultrasound guidance showed partial efface-ment of the lymph node architecture by scattered large cells. Immunohistochemistry showed that these large cells expressed CD30 and CD15 but were negative for CD45.

Questions

1. How do you interpret the histopathology results?
2. What other information would you require in order to fully stage the patient?

Answers

1. How do you interpret the histopathology results?

These cells have the characteristic immunophenotype of the Reed–Sternberg (RS) cell of classical Hodgkin lymphoma.

2. What other information would you require in order to fully stage the patient?

Clinical staging of Hodgkin lymphoma requires a full history, with particular focus on determining the presence of B symptoms (defined as fever ≥38°C, soaking night sweats, or weight loss ≥10% within 6 months), clinical examination, and laboratory workup.

FDG-PET is recommended as part of routine staging at initial diagnosis in conjunction with CT scan. PET-CT is more sensitive than other imaging modalities at detecting disease in unenlarged nodes. Bone marrow trephine biopsy is not indicated in routine staging of clinically localized (stage I–IIA) classical Hodgkin lymphoma, as the risk of bone marrow involvement is <1%.

The patient denied B symptoms and underwent staging including a FBC (Table 26.1) and PET-CT imaging (Fig. 26.1). Increased tracer uptake was seen within the left cervical (21mm), supraclavicular (8mm), high paratracheal (12mm), and bilateral axillary regions (largest 14mm). No extranodal disease was noted.

Table 26.1 Full blood count

	Value in this patient	Normal range
Haemoglobin	12.8g/dl	11.5–16.0g/dl
WBC	9.1×10^9/L	$(4–11.0) \times 10^9$/L
Platelets	193×10^9/L	$(150–400) \times 10^9$/L
Neutrophils	6.97×10^9/L	$(2.0–8.0) \times 10^9$/L
Lymphocytes	1.64×10^9/L	$(1.0–4.5) \times 10^9$/L
ESR	28mm/h	3–9mm/h

WBC, white blood cells; ESR, erythrocyte sedimentation rate.

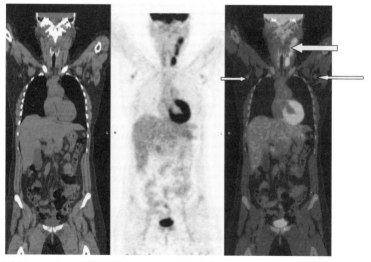

Fig. 26.1 Pre-treatment PET-CT shows activity in left cervical and bilateral axillary nodes (See also colour plate section)

Questions

3. What is the stage of this patient's disease and her risk group?
4. What treatment would you recommend?
5. How would you modify chemotherapy in respect of cytopenias? Would you advise the use of growth factors?

If radiotherapy is included in your management plan:

6. Describe your intended radiation technique and dose.
7. What adverse effects of radiotherapy would you consent for?

Answers

3. What is the stage of this patient's disease and her risk group?

The Ann Arbor staging classification (with Cotswold modifications) is widely used for the staging of Hodgkin lymphoma (Table 26.2). According to this system, the patient should be staged as IIA.

Patients are further classified according to the presence of clinical risk factors. These are broadly similar amongst the main cooperative groups; those used by the influential German Hodgkin Study Group are shown in Box 26.1. With involvement of four nodal areas above the diaphragm, this patient would be classified as having early unfavourable (non-bulky) Hodgkin lymphoma.

Table 26.2 Modified Ann Arbor staging system for Hodgkin lymphoma

Stage I	Single lymph node region (I) or one extralymphatic site (IE)
Stage II	Two or more lymph node regions, same side of the diaphragm (II) or local extralymphatic extension plus one or more lymph node regions same side of the diaphragm (IIE)
Stage III	Lymph node regions on both sides of the diaphragm (III) which may be accompanied by local extralymphatic extension (IIIE)
Stage IV	Diffuse involvement of one or more extralymphatic organs or sites
X	Bulky tumour defined as any single mass of tumour tissue >10cm in largest diameter
E	Extranodal extension or single, isolated site of extranodal disease
A/B	B symptoms—weight loss >10%, fever, drenching night sweats

Source: data from Lister TA et al, Report of a committee convened to discuss the evaluation and staging of patients with Hodgkin's disease: Cotswolds Meeting, *Journal of Clinical Oncology,* Volume 7, Number 11, pp. 1630–36, Copyright © 1989 with permission from the American Society of Clinical Oncology.

Box 26.1 Clinical risk factors in Hodgkin lymphoma

- Large mediastinal mass (at least one-third of the maximum thorax diameter)
- Extranodal disease
- Involvement of three or more nodal areas
- Elevated erythrocyte sedimentation rate (>50mm/h for stages IA, IIA and >30mm/h for stages IB, IIB)

Source: Data from Engert A et al., Reduced treatment intensity in patients with early stage Hodgkin's lymphoma, *New England Journal of Medicine,* Volume 363, Issue 7, pp. 640–52, Copyright © 2010, Massachusetts Medical Society.

4. What treatment would you recommend?

The standard treatment for early unfavourable Hodgkin lymphoma is considered by most groups to be combined modality treatment with four cycles of adriamycin, bleomycin, vinblastine, and dacarbazine (ABVD) (Box 26.2) and 30Gy involved-field radiotherapy.

Box 26.2 The ABVD regimen

- Adriamycin 25mg/m^2 intravenously (IV) on days 1 and 15
- Bleomycin 10U/m^2 IV on days 1 and 15
- Vinblastine 6mg/m^2 IV on days 1 and 15
- Dacarbazine 375mg/m^2 IV on days 1 and 15
- Cycle repeated every 28 days

---

5. How would you modify chemotherapy in respect of cytopenias? Would you advise the use of growth factors?

Treatment should continue unmodified despite low platelet or neutrophil counts, and routine granulocyte colony stimulating factor support is not required.

6. Describe your intended radiation technique and dose.

Radiotherapy should be planned using 3–5mm contiguous CT imaging with appropriate immobilization, including a customized head shell. Volumes should be defined using the ICRU concepts of GTV, CTV, and PTV. Involved-field radiotherapy limits radiotherapy to anatomical nodal regions involved with macroscopic lymphoma and has been adopted as the standard of care in recent trials. Information regarding the location and size of nodes on pre- and post-chemotherapy scans is essential and should be available at the time of planning. The initially involved sites and volumes should be used, tailoring the field borders to the post-chemotherapy volume in areas such as the mediastinum where regression of lymph nodes is readily detected on CT and the sparing of surrounding structures is critical.

For this patient, fields include the whole left neck (upper and lower cervical) including supra- and infraclavicular regions, bilateral axillary lymph node regions, and the upper mediastinal nodes (Fig. 26.2).

Involved-node radiotherapy, in which only the initially involved structures are irradiated, has been proposed. However, for this patient, extensive treatment would still be required; the technique remains unproven and is the subject of current trials.

The standard dose for treatment of macroscopic residual disease is 30Gy delivered over 15 fractions. This patient is not suitable for 20Gy over 10 fractions as she is in the unfavourable risk group.

7. What adverse effects of radiotherapy would you consent for?

Acute reactions are usually mild and transient, and include lethargy, nausea, dermatitis, dry cough, dysphagia, and mucositis. Transient radiation myelopathy

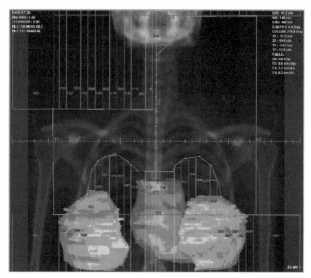

Fig. 26.2 Diagram of suggested radiotherapy field using multileaf collimator (MLC) shaping. Normal structures including the heart (centre) and breasts (left and right) are displayed. (See also colour plate section)

characterized by Lhermitte's sign can occur 6 weeks to 3 months following mantle field irradiation and settles spontaneously after a few months. Radiation myelopathy resulting in paresis has been reported following 30Gy radiotherapy given after standard chemotherapy.

Retrospective analyses of long-term survivors of Hodgkin lymphoma treated over the past three decades have shown elevated relative risks of developing most second malignancies, with breast being of particular concern. This is likely to reflect the long-term consequences of radiotherapy. Due to the involvement of multiple nodal regions the radiotherapy fields required for the patient would be of a size approaching that of a mantle field, and thus extrapolating risk from older trials of extended-field radiotherapy is not unreasonable. A woman treated at the age of 25 with typical mantle fields has an estimated risk of developing breast cancer of 29% by the age of 55; the incidence of other cancers, including those at distant sites, will also be elevated due to low-dose whole-body exposure.

The burden of non-malignant late effects is also significant. Mediastinal irradiation increases the risks of cardiovascular disorder, including myocardial infarction, congestive cardiac failure, and valvular dysfunction, by two- to seven-fold. Twenty-year follow-up of adults treated for Hodgkin lymphoma has also shown a 7% actuarial incidence of non-coronary atherosclerotic disease, such as ischaemic stroke.

After two cycles of ABVD the patient underwent re-staging with PET-CT. This showed no residual FDG uptake but there were persistent enlarged nodes within the cervical and axillary regions consistent with a partial response to treatment. She attends clinic to discuss on-going management but, after hearing about the adverse effects, she declines radiotherapy.

Questions

8. What course of action do you now recommend and how would you counsel the patient?
9. What is her prognosis?

Answers

8. What course of action do you now recommend and how would you counsel the patient?

The results of the Canadian HD6 trial support the use of chemotherapy alone in early stage Hodgkin lymphoma. Patients randomized to ABVD chemotherapy alone had significantly better OS at 12 year than patients whose treatment included subtotal nodal irradiation (94% versus 87%). This was attributed to excess mortality from causes other than lymphoma in the radiotherapy arm. Radiotherapy reduced the risk of relapse by 5%, and since the majority of patients with relapsed disease will be treated with salvage chemotherapy and autologous stem cell transplant, avoiding radiotherapy means accepting an increased risk of requiring more intensive salvage therapy.

This patient had a partial response to treatment after two cycles of ABVD and therefore should be treated with a total of six cycles of ABVD chemotherapy. She should be counselled regarding the increased risk of requiring salvage therapy, which carries significant additional acute and long-term risks, as well as the increased risk associated with the additional anthracycline dose.

9. What is her prognosis?

This patient has an excellent prognosis. The 12-year OS of patients with an unfavourable risk profile treated with ABVD alone in the HD6 trial was 92%, although 16% of patients relapsed over this time and required additional aggressive salvage therapy.

Further reading

Engert A, Plutschow A, Eich HT, et al. Reduced treatment intensity in patients with early stage Hodgkin's lymphoma. *New England Journal of Medicine* 2010; **363**: 640–652.

Ferme C, Eghbali H, Meerwaldt JH, et al. Chemotherapy plus involved-field radiation in early-stage Hodgkin's disease. *New England Journal of Medicine* 2007; **357**: 1916–1927.

Girinsky T, van der Maazen R, Specht L, et al. Involved-node radiotherapy (INRT) in patients with early Hodgkin lymphoma: concepts and guidelines. *Radiotherapy and Oncology* 2006; **79**: 270–277.

Nangalia J, Smith H, Wimperis J. Isolated neutropenia during ABVD chemotherapy for Hodgkin lymphoma does not require growth factor support. *Leukemia and Lymphoma* 2008; **49**: 1530–1536.

Townsend W, Linch D. Hodgkin's lymphoma in adults. *The Lancet* 2012; **380**: 836–847.

Yahalom J, Mauch P. The involved field is back: issues in delineating the radiation field in Hodgkin's disease. *Annals of Oncology* 2002; **13**: 79–83.

Case 27

Solitary plasmacytoma

Isabella Maund and Michael Williams

Case history

A 50-year-old firefighter presented with a 2-month history of progressive lower back pain. Examination revealed no focal weakness of his legs but limited mobility secondary to pain. Sensation was normal and no bladder or bowel disturbance was noted. An MRI scan was performed (Fig. 27.1).

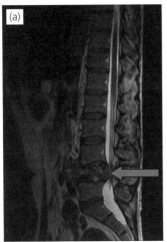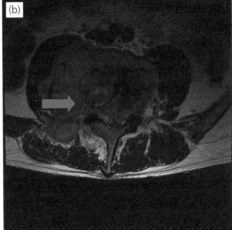

Fig. 27.1

Question

1. Describe the imaging findings in Figure 27.1 and your differential diagnosis.

Answer

1. Describe the imaging findings in Fig. 27.1 and your differential diagnosis.

There is an extensive destructive mass involving the L4 vertebral body, which is fractured and reduced in height. There is a large soft tissue component compressing the theca. No other lesions are obvious within the included images.

The differential diagnosis of a solitary tumour of the spine includes metastatic carcinoma, lymphoma, plasma cell neoplasia, primary malignant spinal tumours such as chondrosarcoma, and benign tumours such as a haemangioma.

*Percutaneous biopsy of the spinal lesion performed under CT guidance revealed a neo-
plasm of dyscohesive cells with eccentric round nuclei. Immunohistochemical staining
was positive for CD138 and kappa light chain, suggestive of a plasma cell neoplasm.*

Questions

2. What staging investigations would you perform?
3. What are the criteria for diagnosing solitary plasmacytoma of bone?
4. What treatment do you suggest if solitary plasmacytoma of bone is diagnosed?

Answers

2. What staging investigations would you perform?

The majority of patients with plasma cell neoplasia will have generalized disease, i.e. multiple myeloma, at the time of diagnosis. A few patients (<5%) will, however, present with truly isolated disease in the form of a solitary bone lesion or rarely a soft tissue mass of monoclonal plasma cells. Staging is required to establish whether apparently isolated lesions are truly solitary and to determine whether there is evidence of bone marrow involvement or end-organ damage, thus essential investigations include:

- FBC
- biochemical screen including renal function and corrected calcium
- serum immunoglobulin levels
- serum and urine protein electrophoresis and immunofixation
- serum free light chain analysis
- bone marrow aspirate and trephine
- full skeletal survey
- MRI of the spine and pelvis.

Standard X-rays have conventionally been used for the skeletal survey and are still employed in current trials. Other imaging modalities, such as whole-body low-dose CT and whole-body MRI, have the advantage of greater sensitivity and have been adopted in many centres. FDG-PET may have a role in selected patients and is useful in the assessment of response following treatment; however, at present PET is not considered a routine investigation.

3. What are the criteria for diagnosing solitary plasmacytoma of bone?

Solitary plasmacytoma of bone is rare, with an incidence rate of 0.34/100,000 person-years. There is a preponderance in men (M:F 2:1), and a median age of presentation of 55 years. It most commonly affects the axial skeleton, especially the vertebrae. Diagnosis requires evidence of a solitary bone lesion which on biopsy shows infiltration by plasma cells, without evidence of systemic disease (Table 27.1).

4. What treatment do you suggest if solitary plasmacytoma of bone is diagnosed?

Radical radiotherapy remains the cornerstone of management of solitary plasmacytoma of bone. In cases of spinal involvement, neurosurgical/orthopaedic opinion should be sought, as there may be a role for surgical intervention in the form of stabilization procedures for loss of structural integrity or neurological compromise. Outside of these indications, surgical intervention is not recommended. Where surgery is required, it should be used in conjunction with radiotherapy; the relative timings of treatments must be decided individually for each patient.

Table 27.1 Diagnostic criteria for solitary plasmacytoma of bone, extramedullary plasmacytoma, and multiple solitary plasmacytomas

Diagnosis	Criteria
Solitary plasmacytoma of bone	No M-protein in serum and/or urine* Single area of bone destruction due to clonal plasma cells Bone marrow not consistent with multiple myeloma (plasma cells <5%) Normal skeletal survey (and MRI of spine and pelvis if done) No related organ or tissue impairment
Extramedullary plasmacytoma	No M-protein in serum and/or urine* Extramedullary tumour of clonal plasma cells Normal bone marrow Normal skeletal survey No related organ or tissue impairment
Multiple solitary plasmacytomas (± recurrent)	No M-protein in serum and/or urine* More than one localized area of bone destruction or extramedullary tumour of clonal plasma cells which may be recurrent

*A small M-component may sometimes be present in blood or urine.
Adapted with permission from The International Myeloma Working Group. Criteria for the classification of monoclonal gammopathies, multiple myeloma and related disorders: a report of the International Myeloma Working Group, *British Journal of Haematology*, Volume 121, pp. 749–757, Copyright © 2003, John Wiley and Sons.

There is limited evidence from small studies that the use of adjuvant chemotherapy may improve the duration of remission and survival. However, at present, there is insufficient evidence to recommend the routine use of adjuvant or maintenance chemotherapy following radiotherapy for solitary plasmacytoma of bone.

The patient was referred to spinal surgeons who recommended L4 laminectomy and stabilization. This resulted in immediate, dramatic benefit in terms of pain control and mobility.

Routine blood tests including FBC, renal function, and calcium levels were unremarkable. Both skeletal survey and bone marrow trephine were negative. Bence-Jones proteinuria was negative with a pre-operative serum M band of 7g/L. A diagnosis of solitary plasmacytoma of bone was therefore confirmed and the patient was consented to undergo radical radiotherapy.

Questions

5. Describe the radiotherapy technique and dose that you would recommend for this patient.

6. What difficulties do you anticipate with delivery of the radiotherapy plan and what late complications should the patient be consented for?

7. What is the prognosis of this patient?

Answers

5. Describe the radiotherapy technique and dose that you would recommend for this patient.

Patients were conventionally planned and treated prone; however, a supine position is acceptable and may be more comfortable for the patient. Appropriate immobilization, including hip fixation and indexed knee rests, is required. Treatments should be planned using three-dimensional CT planning with access to pre-operative MRI images.

An example plan demonstrating the principle of plasmacytoma radiotherapy is shown in Fig. 27.2. The GTV includes the mass and all of the involved bone. This has been grown by 10mm to form a CTV. A 5mm PTV margin has been used as the patient was treated using daily image guidance. The kidney can be seen closely adjacent to the CTV.

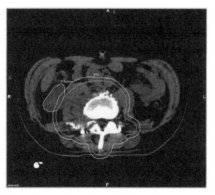 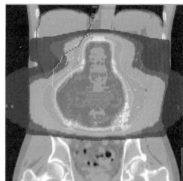

Fig. 27.2 (See also colour plate section)

Tumour bulk has been established as the most important factor influencing local control. Current guidelines recommended a dose of 40Gy in 20 fractions for treatment of solitary plasmacytoma of bone of 5cm or less and that higher doses of up to 50Gy in 25 fractions are considered for tumours of over 5cm.

6. What difficulties do you anticipate with delivery of the radiotherapy plan and what late complications should the patient be consented for?

The OAR most likely to influence radiotherapy delivery in this case is the kidney, and patients should be consented for late effects of renal damage including malignant hypertension, anaemia, and renal dysfunction. According to current recommendations, for partial bilateral kidney irradiation the mean dose should be kept below 15–18Gy and the V20 (the volume of kidney receiving 20Gy) below 32%. Dimercaptosuccinic acid scanning to determine differential renal function may be useful for treatment planning, allowing relative sparing of a dominant kidney if present.

It is estimated that a dose of 50Gy to the spinal cord is associated with a 0.2% risk of myelopathy. Patients should be consented for the potentially severe effects of radiation-induced spinal cord injury including pain, paraesthesia, and paralysis. Other important late effects include vascular complications, including spinal cord haemorrhage, and the risk of radiation-induced secondary malignancy.

7. What is the prognosis of this patient?

Excellent rates of local control in excess of 80% can be achieved with radiotherapy alone. Unfortunately, however, >75% of patients with apparent solitary plasmacytoma of bone will ultimately progress to multiple myeloma after a median duration of 21 months (range 2–135 months). The median OS is 7.5–12 years.

Further reading

Dimopoulos MA, Moulopoulos LA, Maniatis A, et al. Solitary plasmacytoma of bone and asymptomatic multiple myeloma. *Blood* 2000; **96**: 2037–2044.

Hughes M, Soutar R, Lucraft H, et al. *Guidelines on the diagnosis and management of solitary plasmacytoma of bone, extramedullary plasmacytoma and multiple solitary plasmacytomas: 2009 update.* London: British Committee for Standards in Haematology; 2009.

Knobel D, Zouhair A, Tsang RW, et al. for the Rare Cancer Network. Prognostic factors in solitary plasmacytoma of the bone: a multicenter Rare Cancer Network study. *BMC Cancer* 2006; **6**: 118–127.

Lütje S, de Rooy JWJ, Croockewit S, et al. Role of radiography, MRI and FDG-PET/CT in diagnosing, staging and therapeutical evaluation of patients with multiple myeloma. *Annals of Hematology* 2009; **88**: 1161–1168.

Soutar R, Lucraft H, Jackson G, et al. Guidelines Working Group of the UK Myeloma Forum, British Committee for Standards in Haematology, British Society for Haematology. Guidelines on the diagnosis and management of solitary plasmacytoma of bone and solitary extramedullary plasmacytoma. *British Journal of Haematology* 2004; **124**: 717–726.

The International Myeloma Working Group. Criteria for the classification of monoclonal gammopathies, multiple myeloma and related disorders: a report of the International Myeloma Working Group. *British Journal of Haematology* 2003; **121**: 749–757.

Case 28

Clinical trial

Michael Gonzalez, Khurum Khan,
and Bristi Basu

Case history

A 52-year-old woman with stage IIIC high-grade serous-papillary ovarian cancer was referred for consideration of further management having received six lines of treatment over 6 years, including weekly paclitaxel and liposomal doxorubicin, for what had become platinum-resistant disease. A reassessment CT scan showed an increase in the size of her peritoneal lesions with a pelvic mass of 6cm that remained unchanged. Her CA-125 levels had risen ten-fold in 6 weeks from a nadir of 50U/ml (normal <35U/ml). She was asymptomatic. Past medical history included insulin-requiring type 2 diabetes mellitus, an acute myocardial infarction, and essential hypertension. Vascular access was problematic during her last chemotherapy. Since then, she required anticoagulation with low-molecular-weight heparin for a catheter-associated deep-vein thrombosis of the left arm.

Questions

1. What are the treatment options available for this patient?
2. What features of the patient and her disease would it be important to know about in order to consider entry into a phase I study?
3. How should this patient be assessed for eligibility?

Answers

1. What are the treatment options available for this patient?

In view of the platinum-resistant disease and progression after six lines of systemic treatment, this patient no longer has chemosensitive disease. She is asymptomatic but likely to soon encounter complications from disease progression. Options are limited at this stage and good supportive and palliative care is paramount.

Entry into a clinical trial should be considered following careful evaluation. Phase I clinical studies are drug trials that involve the introduction of compounds into patients, either as single agents or combinations, after they have undergone careful pre-clinical evaluation through laboratory experiments in cultured cells and animals (as an initial toxicology screen and to calculate a starting dose). As they may be 'first-in-human' studies, these early phase clinical studies aim to assess safety and tolerability in order to determine a recommended dose to take to phase II trials. Phase II studies then provide an initial assessment of efficacy, subsequently assessed in a randomized setting during a phase III trial. Phase IV clinical studies aim to identify an unexpected toxicity that is likely to be uncommon but potentially serious. However, having had several lines of conventional therapy already, the options of phase II and phase III clinical trials are limited, as in this context standard therapies are quite often compared with the trial medication. Many of these studies also preclude patients who have already received several lines of treatment.

2. What features of the patient and her disease would it be important to know about in order to consider entry into a phase I study?

Specific eligibility criteria should be sought for any individual trial according to those stipulated in published protocols. In general, the following parameters need to be considered:

- Performance status: most studies would require patients to have an ECOG performance status of 0 or 1 at study entry. This patient is asymptomatic and likely to be leading an active life, which is permissive for entry into a clinical study.

- Current symptoms: symptom control should be optimized prior to study entry, for example nausea and vomiting should be controlled before starting an oral drug trial.

- Adequate organ function: depending on how the drug is metabolized, screening for organ dysfunction is required. Organ impairment is likely to affect the safety and tolerability of trial medication, and is particularly important when toxicities of the agent under investigation may worsen organ function.

- Comorbidities: patients with serious and uncontrolled comorbidities, or active infection, are generally excluded from phase I trials. Specific medical conditions might also exclude patients from certain clinical trials, e.g. a patient with a history of arrhythmias or QTc interval prolongation should be precluded from studies on drugs which may have shown a pre-clinical effect on human Ether-à-go-go-Related Gene (hERG) potassium ion channels.

- Potential drug interactions: there is a risk of increased toxicity or diminished drug efficacy with cytochrome P450 (CYP) liver enzymes that are induced or inhibited by concomitant medications.

- Vascular access: many of the novel drugs under investigation are oral agents, but vascular access may still need to be considered since patients on many trials have to provide serial blood samples, e.g. for pharmacokinetic analysis.

- Disease amenable to biopsy: to determine the pharmacodynamic modulation of signalling pathways or to assess treatment efficacy by laboratory analysis of the sampled tissue if this is safe to acquire.

- Expected survival of more than 3 months: this is a generally accepted eligibility criterion for most patients entering a clinical study.

- Patient commitment, but realism: patients can be desperate to continue to be actively managed and treated. They can be desperate not to give up. This patient is very likely to be in this category as she has previously had six lines of treatment and is asymptomatic. However, phase I treatment has no proven efficacy and may just give toxicity and adversely affect her quality of life.

3. How should this patient be assessed for eligibility?

A screening visit is part of the assessment in many clinical trials. At this clinical review, a full history is obtained and physical examination is performed. Careful documentation is important since symptoms and signs that are present at baseline need to be recorded and monitored during the course of the study. Investigations may include:

- Blood tests, including tumour markers to establish that there is biochemical progression, and system-specific investigations to assess organ function. For example, respiratory investigations might involve full lung function tests, whereas cardiac investigations might include an ECG, echocardiogram, MUGA, or Holter monitoring.

- Imaging to confirm the presence of radiological progression. Measurable disease, however, is not always a requirement for clinical trials.

This patient enters a phase III clinical trial evaluating the role of bevacizumab, an anti-VEGF agent, but withdraws from the trial after one infusion because of worsening of pre-existing hypertension. Meanwhile, her daughter, aged 22, is diagnosed with an operable invasive ductal carcinoma of the left breast.

Questions

4. What is the significance of her daughter's new diagnosis?
5. How might this new information influence further management for the patient?

Answers

4. What is the significance of her daughter's new diagnosis?

A thorough family history is important to exclude the possibility of an inherited malignancy. In this case, the occurrence of breast cancer in a first-degree young relative of a patient with ovarian cancer should prompt referral to a specialist in cancer genetics for an assessment to identify whether a germline mutation of the BRCA gene is present. Mutations in the two BRCA genes, *BRCA1* and *BRCA2*, can be of autosomal dominant inheritance but the penetrance is frequently variable between generations. Affected women are at risk of developing ovarian cancer, affected men have a higher risk of prostate cancer, and both genders are at increased risk of developing breast and pancreatic cancers.

5. How might this new information influence further management for the patient?

Tumours in patients who harbour germline mutations of *BRCA1* or *BRCA2* may show increased sensitivity to treatment with poly-ADP ribose polymerase (PARP) inhibitors. BRCA deficiency results in defective homologous recombination repair of damaged DNA. Therefore cancer cells within tumours arising in a BRCA-deficient context are dependent on PARP enzymes which are required for the salvage DNA repair pathway. The observation that single-agent PARP inhibitors could preferentially target cancers harbouring defects in homologous recombination repair of DNA, to achieve profound cytotoxicity within the tumour whilst sparing normal tissue, has provided the first therapeutic example of 'synthetic lethality'. The selective effect of PARP inhibition with drugs such as olaparib (AZD2281) can be observed as a clinical, radiological, and biochemical response in patients who carry a BRCA mutation. The main toxicities of olaparib are nausea, fatigue, and bone marrow suppression, primarily thrombocytopenia. At present, however, PARP inhibitors are not licensed and are only available by enrolment of eligible patients into a clinical study.

The patient commences treatment on a phase I clinical study investigating a novel PARP inhibitor.

Questions

6. What are the aims of a phase I clinical study?
7. What useful parameters are monitored during the course of a phase I study?
8. What factors in the patient history might predict clinical outcome?
9. What other options are available to this woman if she progresses?

Answers

6. What are the aims of a phase I clinical study?

A phase I study is to determine the safety and tolerability of a novel agent or drug combination, as well to establish the dose-limiting toxicity (i.e. the toxicity that is considered unacceptable because of severity and/or irreversibility, limiting further dose escalation). Phase I studies will further indicate the maximum tolerated dose of the trial drug, defined as the highest dose of a treatment that does not cause unacceptable side-effects. Toxicities are recorded using standardized grading criteria, such as the National Cancer Institute (NCI) common toxicity criteria (CTC). Dose-limiting toxicity usually corresponds to NCI CTC grade 3 or grade 4. Preliminary evidence of objective antitumour activity is also reported in phase I studies, for further evaluation in a phase II clinical trial.

7. What useful parameters are monitored during the course of a phase I study?

During a phase I study, and frequently prior to entry, patients provide regular samples of blood and tissue. Frequent visits are required during the early parts of the study when the patient has commenced regular dosing to monitor for toxicities from the trial drug.

Pharmacokinetic tests involve serum assays of blood levels to determine 'what the body does to the drug' in terms of absorption, distribution, metabolism, and excretion. Parameters that are usually defined include the maximum concentration of the drug (C_{max}), exposure to the drug (calculated from the area under the curve or AUC), its half-life ($t_{1/2}$), and clearance.

Pharmacodynamic testing investigates 'what the drug does to the body', for example in terms of nadir counts observed, non-haematological toxicity, molecular correlates of drug inhibition, and imaging end-points such as reduced FDG uptake on PET-CT.

8. What factors in the patient history might predict clinical outcome?

Patient selection for phase I clinical studies can be challenging, because although a predicted life expectancy of more than 3 months is required, accurate assessment of life expectancy is difficult in patients with advanced and treatment-refractory cancer. Performance status can help predict clinical outcome but remains a subjective assessment. The Royal Marsden Hospital prognostic score has been developed and validated as a helpful guide for appropriate patient selection based on a predicted 90-day mortality. To calculate a score out of 3 (minimum 0, maximum 3), one point is added for each of the following features: presence of more than two metastatic sites (one point); serum albumin <35g/L(one point), lactate dehydrogenase higher than the upper limit of normal (one point). A low score of 0 or 1 suggests a favourable prognosis, whereas a high score of 2 or 3 is associated with an unfavourable outcome.

9. **What other options are available to this woman if she progresses?**

Patients who remain well can be considered for another clinical study. Palliative care support should be sought at an early stage.

Treatment and follow-up

The patient was treated with a PARP inhibitor for 2 years. This resulted in a maintained partial response and sustained reduction in CA-125 levels.

Further reading

Ashworth A. A synthetic lethal therapeutic approach: poly(ADP) ribose polymerase inhibitors for the treatment of cancers deficient in DNA double-strand break repair. *Journal of Clinical Oncology* 2008; **26**: 3785–3790.

Cancer Research UK. Phases of trials; 2012. Available at: <http://www.cancerresearchuk. org/cancer-help/trials/types-of-trials/phase-1-2-3-and-4-trials>

Eisenhauer EA, O Dwyer PJ, Christian M, Humphrey JS. Phase I clinical trial design in cancer drug development. *Journal of Clinical Oncology* 2000; **18**: 684–692.

Fong PC, Boss DS, Yap TA, et al. Inhibition of poly(ADP-ribose) polymerase in tumors from BRCA mutation carriers. *New England Journal of Medicine* 2009; **361**: 123–134.

Olmos D, A'hern RP, Marsoni, S, et al. Patient selection for oncology phase I trials: a multi-institutional study of prognostic factors. *Journal of Clinical Oncology* 2012; **30**: 996–1004.

Case 29

A jejunal tumour

Thankamma Ajithkumar

Case history

A 55-year-old man presented with a week's history of melaena. There were no associated symptoms. He had never smoked and was not taking any medications. Further investigations with a barium enema and endoscopies were normal, and his symptom subsided without any intervention.

The patient presented again 8 months later with melaena. His haemoglobin level was 5.1g/dl. He received 10 units of blood transfusion over a period of 3 days. Endoscopies and imaging were normal and he underwent an exploratory laparotomy. At laparotomy, he was found to have an exophytic tumour just distal to the duodeno-jejunal flexure with no other abnormalities in the abdomen.

The tumour was resected. Histopathology showed a 6cm × 4cm × 4cm extramural tumour composed of interlacing fascicles of spindle cells and collagen. The average mitotic rate was 2 per 50 HPF. There was no necrosis. The resection margins were free of tumour. The tumour cells were positive for CD34 and CD117, focally positive for actin, and negative for desmin and cytokeratin.

Questions

1. What is the histopathological diagnosis?
2. How do you estimate the prognosis?
3. Outline your further management.

Answers

1. What is the histopathological diagnosis?

The histopathological appearance is that of a mesenchymal tumour, and the differential diagnoses are gastrointestinal stromal tumour (GIST), leiomyosarcoma, and leimyoma.

GISTs comprise >85% of all sarcomas arising from the GI tract. Around 95% of GISTs express CD117 (a KIT receptor tyrosine kinase), while other malignant mesenchymal tumours are CD117 negative. Before the discovery of CD117, CD34 (a haematopoietic stem cell marker) was the best available diagnostic marker for GIST (60–70% positivity). However, CD34 expression varies according to the location of the primary, with the highest positivity for gastric GISTs (85%) and only 50% positivity for small intestinal GISTs. Some GISTs may show positivity for smooth muscle markers such as actin and desmin. Cytokeratin, an epithelial marker, is usually negative in GIST. Therefore the final pathological diagnosis is a GIST of the proximal jejunum.

GISTs most commonly originate in the walls of the stomach and the small intestine from the interstitial Cajal cells. The presenting features of jejunal GISTs include non-specific abdominal pain, obstruction, or haemorrhage. A pre-operative diagnosis of jejunal GIST is often difficult due to non-specific and variable clinical symptoms.

2. How do you estimate the prognosis?

In 2002, the known prognostic factors were the location of tumour (stomach tumours have the most favourable outcome), size (>5cm was considered malignant), and mitotic rate. Tumours with 0–1 mitoses per 10–50HPF were considered at low risk for metastases and those with >5 mitoses per 50HPF as malignant. The median survival of GIST in the pre-imatinib era was 5 years for resectable disease and 10–20 months for recurrent and metastatic disease.

There a number of tools for estimating the risk of recurrence of GIST such as the National Institutes of Health (NIH) consensus risk criteria, the Armed Forces Institute of Pathology criteria, the modified NIH criteria and the Memorial Sloan-Kettering Cancer Centre (MSKCC) GIST nomogram.

Using the MSKCC GIST nomogram, the 5-year recurrence-free survival of this patient would be 67%.

3. Outline your further management.

This patient had complete resection of a non-metastatic GIST. There was no proven role for any adjuvant treatment and regular follow-up was advised.

During a routine follow-up 4 years later, his liver function tests showed a raised serum ALT and alkaline phosphatase, but he was asymptomatic. An ultrasound of the abdomen showed multiple liver lesions. The CT scan images are shown in Fig. 29.1.

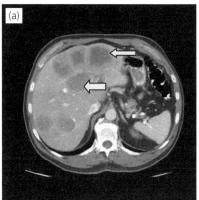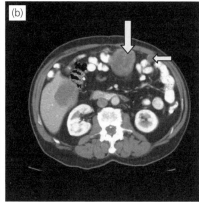

Fig. 29.1

Questions

4. What does the scan in Fig. 29.1 show?
5. If his primary diagnosis of GIST was made only recently, would you advise any adjuvant treatment?
6. Outline your further management.

Answers

4. What does the scan in Fig. 29.1 show?

The scan shows multiple low-attenuation lesions throughout both lobes of the liver. One of the lesions has an enhancing rim (a). No biliary dilatation is seen. There are at least two omental nodules (b). Other images (not shown) showed similar masses in the liver, omentum, and mesentery with no ascites or lymph node mass. The chest was clear. The appearance is suggestive of multiple liver, omental, and mesenteric metastases.

5. If his primary diagnosis of GIST was made only recently, would you advise any adjuvant treatment?

Only 50% of patients with completely resected localized GIST remain recurrence free at 5 years. According to the modified NIH criteria, patients with at least one of the following features are considered as high risk (>15–20% risk of recurrence) and may benefit from adjuvant imatinib:

◆ tumour of >10cm

◆ mitotic index of >10/50HPF

◆ tumour of >5cm with mitotic index of >5/50HPF

◆ tumour rupture

◆ any non-gastric tumour of 2–5cm with a mitotic index of >5/50HPF or 5–10cm with a mitotic index of ≤5/50HPF.

The ACOSOG Z9001 study has reported an improved PFS with 1 year of adjuvant imatinib in patients with GIST of ≥3cm (Dematteo et al. 2009). The recently reported Scandinavian Sarcoma Group (SSG) XVIII trial, which compared 36 versus 12 months of imatinib in high-risk resected GIST, showed that 36 months of adjuvant imatinib resulted in an improved 5-year OS (92% versus 81.7%) and recurrence-free survival (65.6% versus 47.9%) (Joensuu et al. 2012).

According to the modified NIH criteria, this patient has a high-risk resected GIST. However, in the UK, imatinib is not currently approved for adjuvant therapy, though it is recommended according to the National Comprehensive Cancer Network (NCCN) guidelines.

6. Outline your further management.

Since this patient has metastatic recurrence of CD117-positive GIST, the treatment of choice is imatinib 400 mg daily (a TKI). Non-randomized studies of imatinib report a 2-year survival of 78% with a partial response rate of 66% in locally advanced or metastatic GIST. The most common side-effects of imatinib include diarrhoea, fluid retention, nausea, fatigue, abdominal pain, muscle cramps, and rash.

A follow-up CT scan 3 months after starting imatinib at a daily dose of 400mg showed shrinkage of liver, omental, and mesenteric metastases with a marked reduction in the density of liver lesions, and loss of hypervascular rims in some liver lesions (Fig. 29.2). There was no new disease.

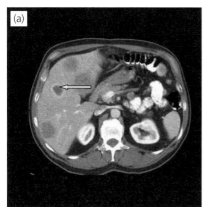 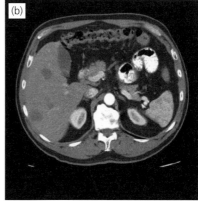

Fig. 29.2

Question

7. What is the significance of the appearance of the scans in Fig. 29.2?

Answer

7. What is the significance of the appearance of the scans in Fig. 29.2?

On the CT scan, among the earliest evidence of treatment response is a decrease in the tumour density (the lesion becoming hypodense). It may take 4–6 months for the tumour to show any shrinkage, and after initial shrinkage the size of the tumour may stabilize. All patients need a scan at 2–3 months after the start of imatinib to rule out any progression.

Three years and 10 months after his follow-up CT scan the patient presented with abdominal cramps. A CT scan showed no change in the size or number of the metastatic lesions in the liver, mesentery, or omentum. There were no new lesions. Some of the liver lesions contained a new soft-tissue component. Figure 29.3 shows that the soft-tissue component in the hypodense lesion has increased from 1.8cm (A) to 2.2 cm (B), and the average attenuation value has increased from 40 to 55 Hounsfield units (HU).

A histopathology review confirmed the previous findings, and also reported DOG1 (Discovered on Gist-1) positivity in the tumour cells. Genetic testing with sequencing of exon 11 of the C-KIT gene has shown a 9 base pair deletion starting at nucleotide 1668.

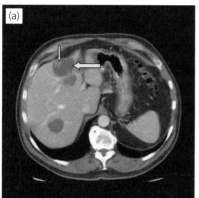 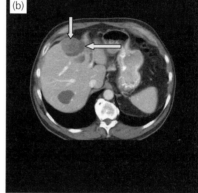

Fig. 29.3

Questions

8. How do you interpret the findings of the scan in Fig. 29.3?
9. What is the significance of DOG1 positivity and the genetic mutation?
10. Outline your further management.

Answers

8. How do you interpret the findings of the scan in Fig. 29.3?

There is a progressive soft-tissue mass in a previously hypodense lesion with an increase in density from 40 to 55HU, an increase of 30%. There is no increase in the overall size of the metastases. According to the RECIST (response evaluation criteria in solid tumours) criteria, which are based on the size of tumour, the disease is stable; however, progression in GIST can manifest as a partial or complete filling of a previously hypodense lesion (Fig. 29.3) or as a hyperdense 'nodule within a mass', without any apparent increase in the size of the pre-existing lesion. These features need to be taken into consideration when assessing disease status in GIST.

Choi et al. (2007) described alternative criteria for evaluating response in GIST and these criteria have been shown to correlate better with survival than RECIST. According to these criteria a 15% reduction in tumour density or 10% unidimensional reduction in tumour size is a better predictor of response.

9. What is the significance of DOG1 positivity and the genetic mutation?

DOG1 is a monoclonal antibody against a chloride channel protein expressed by 95% of GISTs. It has a high sensitivity and specificity, and is also useful in the diagnosis of CD117-negative GIST.

The type of KIT mutation correlates with response to imatinib and survival in patients with GIST. Those with exon 11 mutations have a better objective response (74% versus 44%), and a longer median survival (60 versus 38 months) compared with exon 9 mutations. A meta-analysis has shown that in patients with exon 9 mutations a high dose of imatinib (800mg daily) results in a better PFS and overall response rate (47% versus 21%).

10. Outline your further management.

Though there is some evidence that dose escalation may be an option during progression, particularly in those with an exon 9 mutation, it is not recommended by NICE.

The recommended treatment for this patient is the multi-targeted TKI sunitinib, 50mg daily for 4 of every 6 weeks. The side-effects include fatigue, reaction of the skin on the hands and feet, discoloration of the skin and hair, sore mouth, vomiting, abdominal pain, diarrhoea, mucositis, and hypothyroidism. In imatinib-refractory patients, sunitinib improves PFS compared with placebo (27 versus 6 weeks).

Follow-up and progress

The patient was started on sunitinib and remained well with stable disease after 2 years.

Further reading

Casali PG, Blay JY and the ESMO/CONTICANET/EUROBONET Consensus Panel of Experts. Gastrointestinal stromal tumours: ESMO clinical practice guidelines for diagnosis, treatment and follow-up. *Annals of Oncology* 2010; **21**: v98–v102.

Choi H, Charnsangavej C, Faria SC, et al. Correlation of computed tomography and positron emission tomography in patients with metastatic gastrointestinal stromal tumor treated at a single institution with imatinib mesylate: proposal of new computed tomography response criteria. *Journal of Clinical Oncology* 2007; **25**: 1753–1759.

Demetri GD, Garrett CR, Schöffski P, et al. Complete longitudinal analyses of the randomized, placebo-controlled, phase III trial of sunitinib in patients with gastrointestinal stromal tumor following imatinib failure. *Clinical Cancer Research* 2012; **18**: 3170–3179.

Dematteo RP, Ballman KV, Antonescu CR, et al. Adjuvant imatinib mesylate after resection of localised, primary gastrointestinal stromal tumour: a randomised, double-blind, placebo-controlled trial. *The Lancet* 2009; **373**: 1097–1104.

Joensuu H. Risk stratification of patients diagnosed with gastrointestinal stromal tumor. *Human Pathology* 2008; **39**: 1411–1419.

Joensuu H, Eriksson M, Sundby Hall K, et al. One vs three years of adjuvant imatinib for operable gastrointestinal stromal tumor: a randomized trial. *Journal of the American Medical Association* 2012; **307**: 1265–1272.

Memorial Sloan-Kettering Cancer Centre. GIST nomogram: <http://nomograms.mskcc.org/GastroIntestinal/GastroIntestinalStromalTumor.aspx>

Case 30

The role of specialist palliative care

Nicola Holtom

Case history

A 65-year-old man presented as an emergency with bowel obstruction and hydrone-phrosis having experienced 3 months of rectal pain and altered bowel habit. A rectal tumour was inoperable, and defunctioning ileostomy and ureteric stent insertion was performed.

He was referred for neoadjuvant chemoradiotherapy. He was informed that pre-operative treatment was likely to reduce risk of local recurrence by up to two-thirds. He was undecided whether to proceed with the treatment due to concerns about long-term toxicities. His medications included ibuprofen and paracetamol.

He was referred to specialist palliative care for symptom control and psychological support. He had been feeling overwhelmed since diagnosis, and felt that he was losing control over his life.

His main complaints were:

- *Profuse mucous discharge causing disruption to his life. He was evacuating his bow-els of mucus hourly, day and night.*

- *Exhaustion. Sleep was disrupted by anxiety about rectal leakage. On one occasion he had taken a sleeping tablet and was incontinent of mucous rectal discharge.*

- *Rectal tenesmus pain: a constant feeling of needing to evacuate his bowels associated with intermittent shooting pains in the rectum every few hours.*

- *Psychologically low in mood. He was struggling to adjust to his diagnosis and the effects on his life. The stoma and pads affected his body image. He felt embarrassed by malodour and had withdrawn socially from friends and family. He was mourn-ing his loss of health and role, and felt useless. His general practitioner had pre-scribed citalopram but he had not taken it.*

Question

1. How would you manage his physical symptoms?

Answer

1. How would you manage his physical symptoms?

For management of mucous discharge the options include reduction of peritumour inflammation using prednisolone suppositories (5mg twice a day) or prednisolone retention enema (20mg every 2–3 days). Non-steroidal anti-inflammatory agents (NSAIDs) and octreotide also reduce the volume of discharge. It is important to keep the area dry, protect the skin with barrier ointment, and monitor for fungal infection. Due to the severity of symptoms, octreotide 200µg/24h via a syringe driver was commenced. Within 48h mucous discharge was controlled and he was sleeping through the night. He was subsequently commenced on Sandostatin LAR 20mg subcutaneously every 4 weeks.

With regard to pain management, tenesmus pain has a significant neuropathic component and can be difficult to treat. Tenesmus is likely to increase during chemoradiotherapy and it is important to establish an effective analgesic regime prior to commencing treatment. In accordance with NICE guidelines for the management of malignant neuropathic pain the first-line treatment is to start an opioid and add an antineuropathic agent if the patient develops adverse effects or pain is not controlled. Strong opioids are generally best administered with a non-opioid, and if there is a neuropathic component (as in tenesmus pain) specific antineuropathic agents may be required.

Oral morphine 2.5mg as needed 4-hourly was effective in controlling pain and transdermal fentanyl (12µg/72h) was commenced as this is relatively less constipating than other strong opioids. Tolerance to strong opioids is not a practical problem and physical dependence does not prevent a reduction in the dose of morphine if the pain ameliorates as a result of treatment.

Laxatives should be prescribed routinely for constipation unless there is a reason for not doing so, for example the patient has an ileostomy.

At mid treatment review, he complained of low-grade discomfort in the rectum and was using oral morphine 10mg three to four times a day with good effect.

Question

2. How would you adjust his analgesic medication?

Answer

2. How would you adjust his analgesic medication?

As his pain was opiate-responsive (oral morphine gave total relief of symptoms for 4 h), the fentanyl patch was increased to 25µg/72h.

On completion of treatment he complained of increasing rectal pain, which was only partially relieved with morphine.

Question

3. How would you optimize analgesic control?

Answer

3. How would you optimize analgesic control?

Patients sometimes experience a flare in pain due to treatment. If the pain is responding to opiates the dose should be titrated until symptoms settle. If the pain is not completely relieved with opiates, steroids or NSAIDs can be effective. However, if the psychosocial dimension of suffering is ignored, success will be limited.

Question

4. What psychological support could you offer this man?

Answer

4. What psychological support could you offer this man?

Following holistic assessment, full psychological assessment is needed if symptoms are identified. Symptoms are exacerbated by insomnia, exhaustion, anxiety, and depression. The severity of a symptom is measured by determining the impact that symptom is having on a patient's life.

An explanation of the reasons for the symptoms does much to alleviate the psychological impact. This patient believed that his symptoms would continue indefinitely and was feeling despondent.

Nearly 50% of patients with cancer have a psychiatric disorder as judged by DSM criteria. However, in two-thirds of these patients it is a transient adjustment disorder with depressed or anxious mood.

The first step in helping patients who are feeling overwhelmed by their situation is to enable them to sleep. He was struggling to make decisions because of fatigue but he also wanted to retain autonomy. He described himself as being introspective and prone to worrying but did not feel that he was depressed. Once his symptoms were controlled his mood improved and he completed chemoradiotherapy treatment.

Three weeks later he complained of a 2-week history of increasing rectal pain and offensive rectal discharge. He had become preoccupied and introspective about his situation to the extent that he was unable to engage in family activities. He described anhedonia (loss of pleasure in life), insomnia, anorexia, and weight loss. He was gagging on medication. He was referred to dietetics. He believed his quality of life was so poor that at times he did not want to continue living, although there was no active suicidal behaviour.

Question

5. How would you manage this situation?

Answer

5. How would you manage this situation?

Depression, a sense of hopelessness, and exhaustion, greatly increase the risk of suicide. He felt in despair about his situation and agreed that it was important to optimize physical and emotional well-being prior to surgery. Fentanyl was increased to 50μg/72h and orodispersible mirtazapine 15mg at night was commenced.

Three weeks later he was feeling much more optimistic and was engaged with family life. He was sleeping well with no pain, his appetite had improved, and he had gained a stone in weight.

A re-staging CT scan after neoadjuvant chemoradiotherapy showed response within the primary tumour. A Dukes B adenocarcinoma was completely resected. Post-operatively pain was well controlled and fentanyl was reduced to 37μg/72h.

Three weeks after surgery he was admitted with increasing rectal pain and discharge. CT confirmed a large pelvic abscess, which was aspirated.

His mood was depressed with persistent anxiety and insomnia, being unable to stop thinking about his illness and suffering. He was preoccupied by his symptoms and worries about prognosis. He was losing hope of getting better. Mirtazapine was increased to 30mg and he commenced diazepam 5mg at night. Nasogastric (NG) feeding was commenced due to weight loss.

One month later he was coping well psychologically but experiencing recurrence of tenesmus pain and was using oramorph regularly with only partial pain relief.

Question

6. What are the options for managing his pain?

Answer

6. What are the options for managing his pain?

If pain is only partially relieved with opiates an antineuropathic agent should be added. He was commenced on gabapentin 100mg three times a day. Dose was titrated to 300mg three times a day until pain was controlled.

Two months later he was well. Nasogastric feeding stopped as his target weight was achieved. Diazepam was discontinued and analgesia reduced.

Discussion

Patients completing radical treatment often experience considerable symptom burden (physical and psychological). Thorough holistic assessment will identify their needs.

Patients should be reassured that symptoms can usually be controlled or significantly improved. Instead of expecting immediate, complete relief, symptoms can be improved a bit at a time and much can be achieved with determination and persistence. Never say, 'There's nothing more that I can do'.

Patients will benefit from shared care with specialist palliative care colleagues in seemingly intractable situations.

Progress and follow-up

Eleven months following initial referral he was pain free, psychologically well, and planning a return to work.

Further reading

Harvey M, Dunlop R. Octreotide and the secretory effects of advanced cancer. *Palliative Medicine* 1996; **10**: 346–347.

NICE Supportive and Palliative Care Guidance, 2004 <http://www.nice.org.uk/CSGSP>

NICE. *NICE Clinical Guideline 96.Neuropathic pain*, 2010 http://www.nice.org.uk/nicemedia/pdf/CG96QuickRefGuide.pdf

The National Council for Palliative Care <http://www.ncpc.org.uk>

List of cases by diagnosis

Case 1: Squamous cell carcinoma of unknown head and neck primary site
Case 2: Nasopharyngeal carcinoma
Case 3: Small cell lung cancer during pregnancy
Case 4: Breast metastasis from non-small cell lung cancer
Case 5: Lung cancer in non-smokers
Case 6: Single brain metastasis from breast cancer
Case 7: Breast cancer at a nuclear power station
Case 8: Oesophagus
Case 9: Stomach
Case 10: Neuroendocrine tumour
Case 11: A patient presenting with painless jaundice
Case 12: Colon cancer
Case 13: Rectal cancer
Case 14: Anal cancer
Case 15: Chromophobe renal cell carcinoma in an adult
Case 16: Prostate cancer
Case 17: Testicular cancer
Case 18: Cervical cancer
Case 19: Ovarian cancer
Case 20: Cancer in a renal transplant recipient
Case 21: Melanoma
Case 22: Merkel cell carcinoma
Case 23: Soft tissue sarcoma
Case 24: Bone sarcoma
Case 25: Brain tumour
Case 26: Hodgkin lymphoma
Case 27: Solitary plasmacytoma
Case 28: Clinical trial
Case 29: A jejunal tumour
Case 30: The role of specialist palliative care

List of cases by principal clinical features at presentation (case numbers in italics)

List of cases by aetiological mechanism (case numbers in italics)

Cancer of unknown primary *1*

Genetic mutation *5, 23*

Human papillomavirus *1, 20*

Metastasis *4, 6*

Primary cancer *2, 3, 8, 9, 10, 11, 12, 13, 14, 15, 16, 17, 18, 19, 21, 22, 24, 25, 26, 27, 29*

Radiation-induced cancer *7*

Index